— THE —

WATER
WALKER

A Mother's Resilient Journey of Manifesting
God's Strength to Overcome Life's Obstacles

JULIANNE KIRKLAND

Sorella Enterprises, LLC

inspiredlifementor.com

Designed by: Transcendent Publishing

Edited by: Lori Lynn Enterprises

Cover Photo by: Emily Gearhart

ISBN: 978-1-7354244-0-8

DEDICATION

To my husband Matt and my kids Campbell, Jack, Ashton, Bradlee, Walker, and Meyers for always inspiring me to never give up—no matter how much craziness we go through! And to my dad, for teaching me never to take for granted my ability to choose one thought over another.

ACKNOWLEDGMENTS

I am forever grateful to my family (immediate and extended) for their love, support, and ability to keep me humble.

I want to thank my former business partners Casey Jo and Emily who believed in me and allowed me the honor of helping them to believe more in themselves.

I am grateful for the empowering women in my life (Jennifer Smith, Suzanne Chambers, Marshawn Evans Daniels, Sandra Haseley, Christina Lecuyer, Rachel Luna, Lori Lynn, and Kelly Martin) for "The right word at the right time is like precious gold set in silver. Listening to good advice is worth much more than jewelry made of gold." (Proverbs 25:11-12 CEV®).

I am grateful that these women led by example, as good stewards of their God-given gifts to help others.

I want to thank my mom for reading and editing multiple copies of this book, and all those who read my first few copies and gave me feedback.

I am blessed that my wounds are now scars allowing me to live fully into the best version of myself. And above all else, I am grateful to passionately pursue my calling—to advance the kingdom, be a woman of faith, and add value to others!

CONTENTS

PROLOGUE

Consider it pure joy, my brothers and sisters, whenever you face trials of many kinds, because you know that the testing of your faith produces perseverance.

—James 1:2-3 NIV

I don't know about you, but that verse always seemed easier to say to another person than to accept for myself.

"Consider it pure joy."

Joy?

Trying to apply that verse to my life had me feeling like I had a different definition of joy, or perhaps the trials referenced in the verse were much simpler than mine.

My trials spread out before me like a large body of dark water. A water so cold it took my breath away as I merged deeper in. A water that kept me constantly looking behind and below me, desperate to glimpse what was causing the unrelenting feeling of approaching peril.

Treading the rising water proved a challenge as my body, mind, and spirit had grown weary. My physical body was pushed to the extreme with a high-risk pregnancy. At the same time I was struggling to carry quadruplets to term, I was also watching my father succumb to Alzheimer's, dealing with the betrayal of loved employees, and enduring the failure of the business I had poured my heart into growing. As I wrestled to find the elusive work-life balance, I feared my fragile marriage would shatter.

How was I to consider those trials a joy?

I was a believer, after all; shouldn't that have protected me from enduring so many hard things? Unfortunately, that is not how God works.

Even as a believer, I became uncomfortably acquainted with fear, a sense of overwhelm, scarcity, and depression.

Feelings of inadequacy and confusion became unyielding companions throughout my most trying times.

I thought if I believed more, I would finally experience the incumbent relief from all my hard.

Although God required my faith, it was not for the mere benefit of changing my conditions and circumstances; but rather, for the life-altering enjoyment of changing me.

Noah didn't believe the ark into existence, he got a hammer and got to work.

Was Noah's faith a crucial tool used in building the ark? Absolutely! Did he also have physical tools and help? Absolutely!

I had always heard, "It is the struggles in life that build character." However, I discovered it was the struggles in life that *revealed* my character.

It was the low-tide moments in life that offered a less treacherous terrain for me to catch my breath and think more clearly.

Only in times of focused clarity was I ever able to truly build upon my character.

After all, Noah had to build the ark before it started raining.

I can only imagine if God gave Noah his great commission in this day and age. After hearing from God, he would have FaceTimed with his bestie to get his perspective, then conducted an Instagram poll to see what everyone else thought he should do.

He then would join a Facebook® group of ark builders to get their expert opinions. Next, he would spend countless hours scrolling on YouTube™ to determine the best overall aesthetic for the ark until he would end up stuck, overwhelmed by the increasing rain, standing beside a pallet of wood, holding a hammer—crying out to God for help!

Through the darkest storms and the deepest waters, I would unknowingly develop a process of turning my trials into triumphs. After all, my story is not one of great sadness and trepidation. My story is one of preserving faith, manifesting strength, and learning to walk on water.

In the book of Matthew, we learn the story about Peter stepping out in faith and walking on the water towards Jesus. It was only when Peter took his focus away from Jesus to the storming winds around him that he began to sink. But in that moment of pure dependence and need, Peter cried out, "Lord, save me!"

Immediately, Jesus reached out his hand and caught him. Jesus then responded, "You of little faith, why did you doubt?"

Allowing water to be a metaphor for all life's obstacles, walking on water is a metaphor for manifesting God's strength to overcome those obstacles.

Much like the faith Peter displayed, my journey of walking on water would not be without distraction or "sinking" moments.

My story is real, and turning my storms into a light rain shower for the sake of not offending the clean, seemingly perfect people, would not do God's redeeming power justice.

God loved me just as much when I was in my stormy season, battling depression, questioning my faith, being hot-tempered, and comparing my lack to others' blessings.

He loved me even when I was using bad words in intense situations, or the countless other times I didn't have it all together, just as much as he loves me when I am in my rainbow season, enjoying all the beauty life has to offer.

I believe the depth and variety of ways God shows His consistent love for me is how I am now able to consider my story a joy!

And it began under the most extraordinary circumstances.

CHAPTER ONE

Battling for Babies

When my heart is overwhelmed lead me to the rock that is higher than I.

—Psalm 61:2 KJ21®

The ambulance only used lights, no sirens, to carry me and our four 23-week, unborn babies 100 miles away. We were headed to the best neonatal care hospital in the state of Georgia.

I was an ordinary, young mother battling extraordinary circumstances. The contractions were coming every five minutes or whenever the ambulance hit a bump in the road.

The "what if's" began to overwhelm my thoughts ...

What if we didn't get to the hospital on time?

What if my little boys at home didn't understand why their mommy was being rushed away from them?

I didn't even get to say goodbye or kiss their chubby cheeks. *What if this would scar them for life?*

I shoved my palms into my eyes trying to keep the thoughts

from escaping with my tears. *What if I couldn't do this after all? What if God was asking too much of me?*

* * *

As a young girl with bandages on my knees, a smile on my face, and a bouncing, curly, blonde ponytail, I dreamed of becoming many things when I grew up. A princess, a circus performer, or my favorite (and longest-running dream): a dolphin trainer.

Like I imagine for most, those dreams evolved as I did.

In all of the dreams I had for my life, never once did I dream I would become a mom of six, and I never ... not ever ... had even a fleeting thought that I would have a set of quadruplets.

My first response to the equally stunned doctor was, "Who has four babies?" To which she replied with no words, just head shaking and clasped hands over her mouth.

Although I understood her silence, it was unnerving. True to my personality, I eased the tension with some comic relief. "So, can you tell my husband? Or like, do you have a pamphlet I can give him?"

After moments of nervous laughter (from both of us), the doctor assured me that the odds of all four sacs developing beyond this first appointment were not in our favor.

Sad as that thought was, I felt a wave of comfort knowing I would not likely be having quadruplets. Nevertheless, my husband knew I had gone to the doctor to confirm our positive home pregnancy test.

We had prayed so diligently for this baby.

Six years prior, I was scheduled to have surgery to remove excess endometrial tissue in hopes I would have a better chance of getting pregnant.

Nearly a year after we started trying, the weight of disappointment and the once-a-month, full seven-day reminder that my body wasn't able to do what a woman's body was created to do, was becoming paralyzing.

Thankfully, God was working in the 25th hour. Just before my pre-op appointment, I found out I was pregnant with our first child, our son Campbell.

I did not have one of those "I love being pregnant" kind of pregnancies. Besides the typical morning sickness, I also experienced afternoon sickness, evening sickness, and often late-night sickness.

Just before I was 20-weeks, I began having extreme pain and bleeding. Thankfully, the bleeding was coming from a partial placental abruption instead of a miscarriage, so we carried on, hopeful, but a bit more cautiously.

We began trying to get pregnant with our second child shortly after Campbell's first birthday. We figured if it was going to take another year to conceive, we'd better get on it. Five days before Campbell's second birthday, we welcomed our second son, Jack, into the world.

My second pregnancy was far less dramatic than my first, paving the way for my desire to want a third child in the future.

A couple of years later, we were elated and shocked to find out we were pregnant with twins.

I just knew they would be girls ... I mean, how perfect would our family be? Two beautiful boys two years apart followed by twin girls ... yes, please!

My maternal grandmother was an identical twin and so was my dad! It all fit into a perfect family story; however, the thing I have learned about perfection is that it is actually the lowest standard to reach for because perfection is unattainable. Not for lack of effort, but because perfection does not actually exist.

My idealistic family dream bubble would pop when I went in for my 11-week ultrasound. Having had a placental abruption in the past, and now carrying twins, my doctor wanted to check me a little more frequently.

I always loved hearing the fast flutter of a baby's heartbeat in utero. It filled me with such hope and peace. However, at this appointment, I would experience a whole new set of emotions.

Within a few moments of scanning across my belly, the doctor turned off the sound and switched from the on top of the belly probe to the internal vaginal probe. She said she was having a hard time picking up both babies as they were smaller than she was anticipating.

Naively I thought, "Silly little girls, must be because they are twins."

The doctor picked up on Baby A's heartbeat, no problem. Baby B, however, was silent and much smaller. She concluded that Baby B had died shortly after my eight-week appointment.

Too stunned to cry, I blurted out a series of questions without a single pause for the doctor to respond: Why have I not had any symptoms or bleeding? Would Baby A survive? What happened? How did she die? What will happen to her in my body? What did I do wrong?

The tears came easily now as I listened to her response.

"We never really know what causes a miscarriage early on

like this. In most cases, the fetus has chromosomal issues making it impossible for further development. I cannot be certain if this is the case for you. Your body may absorb the fetus or discard it. Since your babies were not sharing a sac, Baby A should be able to develop normally."

My waterproof mascara didn't stand a chance against the tears steadily flowing as I drove back to work. I felt defeated. Inept. A failure.

I was grateful for the baby remaining but couldn't help feeling I had forever let her down by not being able to carry her sister.

Two weeks passed, and I began to forgive myself and get excited for my baby that remained. I was headed to my follow-up ultrasound appointment only to once again have my bubble burst. Baby A had died, and I was now at a 50% success rate of being able to carry any baby to term.

The depression that followed the miscarriage of my twins was my first experience with the darkness, sorrow, and chest-crushing pressure that would wake me up in the middle of the night.

I allowed myself a full two days after my D&C (the surgical removal of pregnancy tissue) to lie in my bed, heal physically, and begin to heal emotionally and spiritually.

I knew I still had to be mom to my two little boys, for whom I was now even more grateful.

Depression was no place I wanted to linger, but I knew if I didn't allow myself a little time to really feel my emotions and grieve through them, I would be doing myself a disservice.

I would continue to pray for God's mercy as I did not want this failure and loss to be the end of our family story.

Once our six-week recovery time frame had passed after the D&C, Matt and I began trying again to no avail. Months later I would learn that on top of my PCOS (polycystic ovarian syndrome) and endometriosis, I also had fewer eggs in my ovaries than a woman at my age should have.

I was only 29, but my ovaries looked 20 years older. I pleaded with Matt to agree to fertility treatments or IVF (in-vitro fertilization). After many conversations and a lot of prayer, he agreed to one round of Clomid and an IUI (intrauterine insemination, a.k.a. the turkey baster).

By God's grace, our prayers were answered, and our world was turned upside down!

Since our doctor had no interest in giving me a pamphlet or telling my husband he was going to father four more, I had to do it.

I wish I could say that I created a perfect candlelit dinner of his favorites or put together a clever scavenger hunt but, alas, I was still trying to wrap my head around the news.

I had no room for creativity.

As Matt heated up his dinner in the microwave, I casually walked into the kitchen with the ultrasound photos.

"I had my appointment today," I said.

"Yeah, and how did that go?" He turned from the microwave to see my reaction.

"Well … there are four!" I said.

"Four what?" he asked.

"Four babies! Look!" I showed him each individual baby sac.

Without a word, he continuously nodded his head and turned back to face the microwave. The only sound was the soft deep hum of the oven and it felt like it was penetrating my soul.

"Ok ... well ... I'll be over here on the couch if you have any questions," I said.

Matt had only ever wanted one child. When I brought up wanting a second child, he said he didn't think he could love anyone else, that Campbell and I had his whole heart. But the moment he held Jack, his heart made room.

I knew it would be hard. Heck, having two kids was challenging. It elevated our family dynamic and required a new level of organization to maintain sanity. But having four more? At the same time? I had no idea what would be required, not only for sanity but also for sheer survival.

All I knew about being pregnant, being a mom, and being a wife—all I knew about myself and my faith would be forever changed.

✳ ✳ ✳

At 23-weeks pregnant, I started having contractions early in the day and called my sister Karen to ask her to take me to my doctor's office. Since I had been on modified bed rest for the past two weeks and often got lightheaded, I was no longer allowed to drive.

Karen recommended I call my doctor first and let them know what was going on. So, being the always cooperative younger sister that I am, I agreed.

The doctor told me to err on the side of caution and go straight into L&D (Labor and Delivery) at the hospital and she would be there shortly.

The car ride to the hospital came with mixed emotions.

My palms were sweaty, I had an annoying case of dry mouth, and the contractions were still coming. My brows remained furrowed even as I tried to make jokes to hide how scared I was.

My sister laughed appropriately, partly because she understood the severity of the situation and she didn't want to let on that she was nervous too, and partly because, well, I am just funny.

Even though my thoughts were trying to explore every possible outcome, and process a variety of emotions, I still had a sense of peace.

Way, way, way, deep down, I was at peace. I knew I would not be delivering these babies today. God had given me that "peace that passes understanding" (Phil. 4:7 adapted).

Yet I also knew that I didn't know what was going to happen. My mind was at war with my spirit as the contractions continued.

My doctor had already called to let L&D know I was coming, so getting into a room was a breeze. The two hospitals in Athens, where I lived at the time, had been rehearsing my babies' arrival before this day had come.

Once news spread that I'd chosen not to reduce my babies down to two, the hospitals were on high alert. I had already met with the head of the Neonatal Intensive Care Unit and discussed our plan of action for when the delivery day would come; however, we had not discussed the babies coming so early.

By many doctors' standards of practice, 23 weeks is not even considered a viable gestation for survival outside of the womb. All this to say, when I arrived, there was no hesitation in getting these contractions under control. I was immediately monitored and put on fluids and magnesium, aka satan's drug. Okay, so it is not really referred to as "satan's drug," but it should be. The body experiences an inferno of what I can only imagine hell to be.

Although my eyeballs felt like they were on fire, the contractions had calmed down and spaced out. I had called my husband and told him not to worry. I was fine, and these babies were not going to be born today.

I naively assumed that once the contractions stopped, I would be allowed to go back home, so Matt remained at work. I was growing very confident that I would be released, so I asked Karen to go grab lunch for me from my favorite little café that just so happened to be right across the street.

After she left, the nurses informed me that I was not allowed to eat, just as a precaution, in case I were to have a C-section. Typically, I am a very cooperative patient; however, I had been five hours without food!

Some may say, "Five hours? No big deal!"

To that, I say, "Hah!" Even when I'm not pregnant, I don't like to go more than three hours without food. And not only was I pregnant—I was pregnant with FOUR babies!

So, yes, I snuck bites of my favorite chicken salad whenever the nurse would walk out of the room. I was confident my babies weren't coming, and I was starving.

Thankfully, against my Maternal Fetal Medicine (MFM) doctor's opinion, the head neonatologist made the call to go ahead with the steroid shot for the babies' lungs. He viewed my babies as babies and not as fetuses that weren't yet viable. He would do everything in his power to see they had a shot at life outside the womb if the occasion called for it. This was a sentiment that had not been common during the early part of my pregnancy.

* * *

When I first found out that I was pregnant, the doctor doing the ultrasound was just as surprised as I was. She counted two sacs right away ... then, as she moved the wand, she counted three ... then four!

She ran out of the room and grabbed another doctor to come help her count. Here was my doctor, needing help to count to four. If I wasn't so terrified at that moment, I would have found the irony of it all to be funny.

After four sacs were confirmed, the conversation followed about the likelihood that all four would not develop.

I left the appointment shocked, nauseated, lightheaded, amazed, scared, excited, and feeling confident that, at most, we would have triplets.

My confidence grew at my next ultrasound when only three heartbeats could be located. I was sad to a degree, but the overwhelming relief of knowing there would be just three took over. I knew triplets would be tough, but I felt we could handle triplets.

Just one week later, a fourth heart ... beat! And I knew the only way we could handle quadruplets was with God. Each weekly ultrasound that followed was met with anxiety, disbelief, amazement, and physical shaking—not a slight hand tremble, but literal knee-knocking, arm-spasming, body-rocking shaking.

I kept anticipating bad news. I kept waiting to hear only three or two were developing.

Unresolved guilt and sadness still lingered from the twins' miscarriage the year before.

As the weeks progressed, the fear grew stronger. I was able to feel these babies moving much earlier than I could with my first two pregnancies, and although my fear of losing them was, at times, intense, my love for them grew even more so.

At 15-weeks gestation, I was sent to my MFM doctor, who specializes in high-risk pregnancies. The last time my MFM had seen quadruplets was 23 years prior when he was in medical school.

After the long ultrasound, I realized two things: One—I should have invested in the company that makes ultrasound gel with as much as the nurse had to use! (Thankfully, this particular office warmed their gel.) And two—at my next appointment, I needed to be sure to completely empty my bladder beforehand.

Watching my MFM scratch his head in amazement, then close his eyes and firmly rub his fingers slowly up and down between his eyes and his forehead, was unnerving.

I began to chew on my lower lip and look for reassurance from my husband, yet Matt sat wide-eyed, staring at the screen that still held the black and white image of our four little figures.

My doctor took a deep breath followed by a loud sigh. I could feel my heart in my throat as he began to speak.

"Carrying more than two babies at once is never easy, and although everything looks great at this point, that could all change. I would highly recommend you reduce down to two."

I couldn't breathe.

I held my hands together so tightly my fingers turned white. It took all the strength I had to interrupt him in a kind way. "No, no thank you, we will not be doing that." I finally managed to swallow when he interrupted me right back.

"I heard what you said, but I'm going to finish telling you why I think you need to reduce down to two."

My head began to spin and my ears started ringing. I was watching his mouth move, but I could hear no words over my own forced exhaling through my pursed lips. When he finished talking, I rolled my shoulders back, took a deep breath, looked him in his eyes, and said, "No thank you! We will NOT be reducing our babies."

"Well ... okay," he said after an exaggerated long pause. Then he began to tell us stories of how he had been amazed in the past at what a woman's body can do and that I would be closely monitored by his office and my regular OB to ensure the best outcome.

✳ ✳ ✳

Continuing to sneak bites of chicken salad between nurses was lightening my mood and, although satan's drug still burned in my veins and my left hip was sore from a steroid shot, I felt better.

Hopefully, the contractions would remain at bay and the babies wouldn't make their debut until many weeks to come. I would be getting to go home soon. That was my expectation ... until my OB doctor came walking in.

She dragged the cold wooden chair across the overly clean floor (creating a sound that grated on my nerves worse than nails on a chalkboard) up to the foot of the bed, where my newly pedicured toes, painted with three blue balloons and one pink balloon, poked out from under the stiff bed linens.

She took a few deep breaths and said she was elected to be the one to tell me the news.

The news ... what news?

I felt as though everything was fine: the contractions were few and far between, the babies' heartbeats sounded strong and stable, and I was no longer hungry.

Why was my doctor pale and her voice shaky?

I found myself struggling to swallow as she proceeded.

Apparently, while I was sneaking my lunch, my OB, along with the head neonatologist, my MFM doctor, members of the board, and the hospital's attorneys were deciding my fate and the fate of the babies nestled inside me.

My OB explained that, although she didn't feel as if the babies were coming today, the hospital did not feel comfortable with the slim possibility of having four extremely premature babies born there. They were sending me, via ambulance, to a hospital that had a higher-rated NICU and would thus be better equipped to care for my babies.

I would need to remain there until I delivered. I don't think I blinked for an entire minute. After going over the logistics of it all, I said I would do whatever was best for my babies. I began to adjust my stiff sheets to free my sweaty legs and asked if I would be leaving for Augusta later in the evening. To which my doctor replied, "No, now!"

What did she mean, NOW?

My sister had just left to go pick her kids up from school because we thought for sure the babies weren't coming, and I was confident I would be released later that evening!

I was in full-on panic mode, but as my OB walked out of the room, in walked my friend with two large bags of Swedish Fish.

Typically, her smiling face and Swedish Fish can turn around any unfavorable situation; however, this time, I was only able to muster a slight side smile, before my eyes filled.

I knew if I blinked, I would no longer be able to contain my tears. Thankfully, my friend understood the language of sobs and snot. A half a box of tissues later, we both got out our phones and started calling family to try and get the logistics figured out.

How would Matt get down there? Who would watch over our two boys? How would I get my stuff? How much stuff would need to be packed if I was not able to come home until the babies were born? The peace I had felt earlier was being shoved aside by my fear of the unknown.

The icebox ambulance was full. Two EMTs plus their trainee, a neonatal nurse, an OB nurse, and a respiratory therapist crowded in with a very pregnant me!

After being hooked up to satan's drug, my body had been internally boiling for the last several hours. It was a relief to breathe cool, fresh air as I was being wheeled out to the ambulance, and just as refreshing when I entered the crisp, cold air in the mini-hospital on wheels.

I don't know if all ambulances are kept cold, or if mine was cooler because of the number of people traveling, but I was grateful, nonetheless. As I was being loaded, I made an agreement with the driver. I wouldn't have my babies in the back of his ambulance if he would navigate our road trip safely and get me to the hospital as soon as possible.

We both kept our end of the bargain that night. I am beyond

grateful for the encouraging crew that traveled with me. They could see my nerves were getting the best of me. The tears were falling, I didn't want to be 100 miles away from my husband, my boys, my family, my church, my team at work, my friends—my whole support system.

How would I be able to do all this on my own?

The ambulance crew assured me that the decision was made to ensure the best outcome for my unborn babies. A point made that I couldn't argue, no matter how inconvenient and life-altering it all was.

As much as I enjoyed believing in the illusion that I was in control, I prayed that I would get out of my own way and let God be in control. Arriving at the hospital, I had no idea how bad things were about to get.

CHAPTER TWO

Lonely

When you go through deep waters, I will be with you.

—Isaiah 43:2 NLT

The overflow room that I shared with three other women was miserable. All that separated me from my laboring neighbors were two sheets, one that hung a child's arm's length away from the right side of my rock-hard, break-away bed, and the one that hung at the foot of my bed.

These barriers were so close and so thin, I could have literally pointed my toes and cut a hole in the sheet. Although I was in the corner, the smallest space available, I was beyond grateful I had the only window.

A doctor was finally able to make her way to me to check to see if I had dilated, but because she was pushed for time, she did not choose to break away the bottom part of the bed to put me in stirrups, instead she had me ball up my fists and shove them under my hips.

Despite the IV ripping through the vein in the crease of my wrist, I lifted my hips as high as I could. Because my cervix is high and tilts back, she had to insert her entire hand to see if I was dilated. I begged her to stop, gasping for breath through my nose, only to exhale in desperate screams for her to please stop!

I could no longer contain my tears. I had not dilated, but after the exam, my contractions took an angry turn, and I was placed, once again, on satan's drug.

Eyes on fire, I slowed my breathing, turned to my left side, and tried to fall asleep ... that was until the snapping started. Not only would I have a roommate that would snap and yell in her foreign language, but I also had a roommate that brought her posse with her, pulled back the curtains, and had some unspeakable bathroom escapades.

There is no beauty in laboring! I cannot fault her for what her body was going through; however, I can fault her for keeping the *only* bathroom occupied. She would keep the door open so she could talk to her friends while using the bathroom.

I shoved a blanket over my ears, closed my eyes, and prayed I would be able to hold my bladder until after she had been moved to a delivery room. I feared I was only a thin sheet away from hearing a total stranger give birth!

I had just begun to fall asleep when the commotion of her increasing contractions jerked me back into reality. Soon, by the grace of God, she was moved to a private room.

After that, sleep came easy ... until the smell of hospital-grade floor cleaner began to singe my nose hairs. I pulled a corner of the blanket over my nose and continued to breathe through my mouth.

Then there was the woman who seemed to be living out her very own soap opera with her "baby daddy" (her words not mine) over the phone. But that wasn't the worst part.

This particular woman was having to measure and store her urine output, which means she had a container placed between the seat of the toilet and the base to collect any and all urine. No big deal ... except that we all had to share one bathroom, and she refused to move her container.

Every time I made a trip to the bathroom, I had to call the nurse to come take care of her container. The nurse explained to her that all she had to do was pour her container into the specified jug or call a nurse to assist. Again and again, I had to call a nurse when I reached the bathroom.

Leaning on my IV pole while the nurse handled the urine, my exhaustion was taking up the residence of where my patience typically resides. When I rolled back to my bed I heard her chewing me out to whomever she was talking to on the phone. The "Julie" in me began to boil to the surface, and I had the desire to throw her urine container all over her if she left it again.

✳ ✳ ✳

I often refer to my temper, or that less than wonderful side of my personality, as the "Julie" in me. I didn't used to be that way. I rarely had a temper. I grew up as "joyful Julianne!" I was happy-go-lucky and could find the fun and humor in anything. It helped, too, that I was funny myself.

Yet something shifted when I grew up, as I can imagine it does for many. When I was young, I let all my positive emotions lead me. You see, I believe in the "Fruit of the Spirit" from the Bible, where the fifth chapter of Galatians verses 22-23 (adapted) describes it as "love, joy, peace, patience, gentleness, kindness, faith-fulness, goodness, and self-control."

However, the only thing I am perfect at is being imperfect. I strive to walk in faith and submit to the Spirit, but I falter. I'm as human as they come. As I have gotten older, my less than positive emotions can get the best of me. Anger, fear, depression, anxiety, doubt, and selfishness take over, and I have to intentionally change the course of my thoughts. I have found that when I change my thoughts, I change my actions, and by changing my actions, I change my behavior.

✳ ✳ ✳

I did not end up having to dump urine on my neighbor. Thankfully, I was able to fall asleep.

A few hours later, I would be moved to a private room. Privacy was beautiful. I had never been so grateful to lie on a hospital bed. For 46 hours, I had been on a hard break-away bed. I had been uncomfortable for so long, it actually hurt as my muscles began to relax. I didn't know it at the time, but it would be the first of several times my body would feel like it had been through war.

I would remain in the hospital for what seemed the longest seven-day stretch I could remember. It was like the week of Christmas, filled with slow anticipation, but without all the excitement.

The most excitement I experienced was the non-stress test performed twice a day. No big deal for the babies, but getting four monitors on and positioned correctly to be sure they were picking up all four babies' heartbeats took at least thirty minutes, often requiring me to hold a bizarre body position.

Although he was no Santa, I did look forward to my new Maternal Fetal Medicine doctor's rounds each morning. Dr. Browne was a ray of sunshine compared to my last MFM doctor. From the first moment I met him, he was positive, uplifting, and determined to get me and my babies to the finish line, which we had projected to be 28 weeks or beyond.

He referred to my babies as "babies" and not "fetuses" and reminded me to think in hope instead of fear. He was forthcoming about our obstacles but presented them to me in a way that was encouraging. He wanted me to understand that with every week that passed my risk of certain pre-term issues would decrease.

Out of the fifteen or more preemie baby health issues dis-cussed, those that occupied most of my thoughts involved breathing, the brain, and the stomach. My fingers cramped and my eyes burned from the continuous Googling of all the possible ways my pregnancy and birth could go wrong.

I stayed calm and encouraged whenever Dr. Browne and his team visited. Because they believed in me and the possibility of a positive outcome, I grew more confident and hopeful as well.

However, once they left, I was alone with my imagination to keep me company and Google™ to ask my questions. As the hospital room walls closed in, my imagination was anything but a friend.

Thankfully, by the end of the week, I was informed that I would get to leave the hospital but would remain on the hospital campus at the brand new Ronald McDonald House (RMH).

* * *

Two years prior, when my oldest son was just four years old, his appendix ruptured. He was transported to Children's Hospital of Atlanta, where he spent 10 days battling high fever and non-stop diarrhea. He was on IV medications, fluids, and eventually had to have a PICC line put in due to lack of nutrition.

When his fevers would spike, the nurses would have to strip him down and place cold rags under his arms, on his head, and around his feet. Watching your child suffer and not being able to do anything is a debilitating feeling.

I remained with Campbell while Matt traveled back and forth from home. I remember being so grateful that our second son Jack, who was two at the time, had a happy, go-with-the-flow personality. It helped ease my guilt in being away from him.

By day four, though, I asked Matt to bring Jack to the hospital to visit. Thankfully, that night we were approved to stay at the nearby Ronald McDonald House (RMH), which provides free room and board to families whose children are in the hospital.

I was so excited not only to see Jack, but I longed for a hot shower and a bed to sleep in. I had been sleeping in the big chair next to Campbell's bed. I would angle the chair so I was able to put my feet up on the bottom corner of Campbell's bed, and then slept hard in the one-hour increments between the changing of Campbell's diaper (which he had to wear because he was too weak to get up to use the bathroom) and the changing of his medicines.

The thought of a good night's sleep energized me that entire day. Matt stayed at the hospital with Campbell while I took Jack to the RMH. We played in the kids' area together, ate dinner, and got settled into our room.

The RMH was beautiful. I felt like I was at a hotel. Jack watched cartoons while I took my long-awaited, and much-needed, hot shower! We cuddled up tight in the bed and sleep came faster than I could close my eyes.

Not even an hour later I awoke to the increasing body temperature of my two-year-old. I checked his forehead and, sure enough, he felt hot. I moved him to the other bed in the room and placed a cool cloth on his head.

I set my alarm for 30 minutes so I could check on him. I closed my eyes, but when the alarm went off, I struggled to get them open again.

I took a deep breath and went to Jack's bed. He was on fire! His lips were like rubies and his cheeks looked rug-burned. I had NOTHING with me to give him. I didn't even have a car to put him in to go get medicine.

I searched through my purse and found a Tylenol bottle. I

knew I couldn't give him one of my pills of Tylenol, but I also knew I needed to do something. He was miserable and let out soft whimpers while he slept.

I bit off the end of my Tylenol pill and crushed it up using the cap of a pen. I put it in the sip or two that was remaining in my water bottle and tried to get him to drink. No luck. He cried and threw his head back, resulting in the remedy going all over his pillow.

I bit off the second end of the pill, crushed it, and then decided to rub it on his gums.

(Months prior, in one of our monthly personal development meetings, one of my employees was talking to me about her past. She revealed to me how she used to do drugs. Her favorite was the "nummies." That is when she would put the crushed up drug of choice on her gums and receive the high, without having to snort it up her nose. God sure redeemed that conversation. It worked like a charm.)

I remained by Jack's side, waking every other hour to check on him. By morning, the fever was back and I was able to get in touch with Matt to pick up some children's ibuprofen before he came to pick us up. Jack was taken back home to our doctor and was diagnosed with the flu.

Although my stay in the Atlanta RMH was short and didn't end in the way I expected, relief washed over me knowing that the Ronald McDonald House I would be staying at this time (in Augusta) would be within walking distance of the hospital. An appreciated and somewhat necessary perk, considering I had no car. I was also grateful I would be in a more home-like atmosphere instead of having to stay in the hospital until the babies were born.

I was the very first resident at the new Ronald McDonald House and, therefore, my move-in day was captured by the media. I felt like a less-than-glamorous celebrity as I was wheeled from the hospital to the RMH with cameras rolling, pictures being taken, and the entire staff with volunteers there to greet me and help me get settled in my room.

The main floor housed the lobby, kids' play area, dining area, and kitchen, along with two rooms that were reserved for children who need special air-quality-controlled rooms. My room was located on the second floor, a few feet away from the elevator. I was on stair restriction and had to remain on modified bed rest (which allowed me to be able to get up to use the bathroom, take a shower, and walk downstairs to the kitchen long enough to get something to eat.)

As the weeks crept by, my room filled with more and more of my stuff from home. Every Friday, Matt would leave work early and bring the boys down to visit. We hooked up a game system, we had toys, and Matt bought a shelving unit that I could put my food items on. For all intents and purposes, we had made 150 square feet our home away from home.

Sundays became the hardest day for me because I knew that after lunch, a big part of my heart was leaving. Matt was so diligent to make sure all my clothes and linens were washed and in their appropriate places, my groceries were stocked, and I had plenty of *my* toilet paper (the good kind, multi-ply, with grooves and lotion).

I cried every time they left and prayed that God would watch over my family as they traveled back home.

Mondays came too soon but passed equally so. I typically had my check-up and ultrasound with Dr. Browne on Tuesdays, and the anticipation of seeing my babies' little faces and finding out how much they had grown, helped pass the time.

Plus, I looked forward to the short walk to Dr. Browne's office. Being outside helped restore my soul. Resting up in my room with books, TV, my computer, and a window as my only means of interaction with the outside world was hard on me.

It was the middle of winter, and looking outside at the bare trees and wilted leaves where flowers had once been was depressing; however, once I was outside I could breathe in the cool, crisp air.

Every so often, the clouds would part just enough for a ray of sunshine to hit my face. I would stop mid-stride and soak in the sunshine, deep breaths and all. I'm sure to all those who passed by, I seemed nuts. On a few occasions, I even had people walk up to me and ask if I needed help getting to the hospital.

A few hours after returning to my RMH home from each appointment, depression would kick in. Seeing my family was still days away and there I was, alone! I would blog, read, chat with friends or family and watch TV, but I felt alone.

I wanted to sleep but couldn't. Lying down was uncomfortable and awkward, and because Baby D was up under my ribs, it took my breath away every time he moved. Sitting was worse. I hated the feeling of my belly resting on part of my thighs just above my knee.

The only comfortable position involved the strategic placement of eight pillows: three behind my back and neck, one on each side, two under my knees, and one wedged between my belly and thighs. This position was never a quick one to get into, but once accomplished, and after my breathing slowed, it was glorious—until ten minutes later when I would have to go pee.

The constant getting up to go to the bathroom was annoying, but it occupied my mind as I would make it into a game for myself. I would try to watch a full 30-minute show or read three chapters of my book before getting up. Simple right?

Wrong!

I often had to get up to pee every commercial break, so this was indeed a challenge. Drinking at least a gallon of water a day was tough in the beginning, but once I was used to it, it was easy! I took drinking my gallon a day seriously, as doing so supplied my babies with their needed fluids and helped keep Braxton Hicks contractions at bay.

Plus, filling up my jug several times a day allowed me the excuse to ride the elevator down to the kitchen, get some ice, and refill my water. The RMH had the best ice. It was the small cylindrical kind, great for crunching. When you are alone, you have to find joy in the little things, such as small crunchy ice and bathroom games.

By Thursdays, the anticipation of my husband and boys coming to visit fueled my spirit. We Skyped every night, but knowing I would get to hold, squeeze, and kiss their sweet faces kept a smile on my face and a hop in my step! However, not a literal hop … as I was huge, and my feet were swollen. Picking my feet up off the ground, in a non-shuffle form, was an act of God!

I also had two cousins (on opposite sides of the family) who lived near the hospital and would often bring me lunch and stay to chat for a bit. I was so grateful when one of my cousins brought me back to her house one Sunday evening for a wonderful dinner and a hot bath in her *huge* tub.

One of the hardest things about the RMH was the bathroom. Although nice, it was not built for hugely pregnant women. The standard tub/shower was hard to get in and out of, and because so many guests were in the house, if you tried to take a bath or shower during typical bathing hours, you quickly ran out of hot water.

Another challenge I was excited to overcome was figuring out the best time to bathe. For a shower, it was 6:30 a.m. For a bath, it was 10:30 p.m., and even then, I could only get enough hot water to cover the tops of my shins.

Because the tub was more narrow than wide, I had to sit straight up with my legs straight forward. I would take a washcloth, roll it up, and wedge it under my belly because the feeling of my belly resting on my thighs was one of the most annoying sensations I had ever experienced.

Getting out of the tub was a strenuous and hilarious feat. I couldn't help but laugh at my grunts and exasperated exhalations as I tried to maneuver my way to a standing position. Then came even more laughter as I tried to dry myself.

I would take a towel, and in true old school, boy's locker room fashion, I would spin my towel round and round and whip it around my leg as I pulled it upwards. Surprisingly, this method worked quite well in drying areas I could no longer reach.

By the time I managed to get my body mostly dry and waddle back to my bed, I would have to plop down for a few minutes of rest before struggling to get my pajamas on.

Bathing and dressing had me exhausted! I knew it was necessary, but I struggled to convince myself it was actually worth it!

Then, I had the ordeal of getting my pillows accurately placed, making sure I had the TV remote, phone, and my water within reaching distance before I could melt into my bed.

Then within minutes, I would have to pee again. So taking a hot, full bath, in the early evening with scented bath salts at my cousin's house, felt like a glorious time.

I remember how rolling onto my side, allowing the water to help support my belly, brought tears to my eyes. I realized at that moment how much I took for granted in my everyday, pre-pregnancy comforts.

I cried out to Jesus and thanked him for the privilege of being able to carry four babies for as long as I had, and I cried even more when I thanked him for the blessing of hot, clean, running water and a bathtub large enough to float in.

God asks of us in 1 Thessalonians 5:18 (KJV): "In every thing give thanks." Although I'm sure it seemed small to the Almighty, his mercy and grace for this tub experience were huge to me!

I am never amazed at the seesaw of my faith in my circumstances. I can rejoice in a home-cooked meal and a bath one day, yet the next, I can slip into the darkness. Living in almost total isolation, the darkness threatened to creep in daily.

Although I was carrying four babies and would have sporadic visitors throughout the week, I battled loneliness. The solitude was debilitating.

I would keep all the lights on to help combat the dark thoughts that crept in like the tide (the kind where you think you have picked a good elevated spot on the sand, you finally fall asleep under the warm sun, only to frantically be awakened to the ice-cold waters soaking you, your towel, and all your stuff).

Once a week, I would have an emotional meltdown while talking to my husband on the phone. I would beg him to let me come home! I promised I would keep the babies in until 32 weeks if he would just bring me home.

We both knew I was where I needed to be, but every week he patiently and lovingly reminded me why I needed to stay. Never once was he annoyed with my sobbing, nor did he tell me to stop and toughen up. He let me have my moment and assured me how much I was loved and how much he appreciated what I was doing for our babies. Such a simple act made a huge difference.

Only twice were our roles reversed and he needed my support and encouragement. In the blink of an eye, he had been practically thrown into single-parenthood. I typically ran the house. I set the routine for school and all that involved. I fed the animals, I managed the extracurricular activities, did the grocery shopping and the laundry—I ran the house!

Did I do it perfectly? No. Did it work well for our family? Yes. Without me home, he missed me.

Yes, he was now aware of all that I did, but more than that, he missed his partner. He missed me reaching over in the middle of the night to hold onto his arm. He missed kissing me goodbye before he left for work. He missed talking to me about his day and asking about mine and the boys' day. He missed his wife! And although he had our boys, he felt alone.

Before this experience, I had yearned to have time alone. Being a mom of two kids, I rarely went to the bathroom by myself, but being secluded in a small room, two hours away from family was not at all what I meant by wanting some *alone time*.

I was 27-weeks pregnant and my isolation was more than geographical seclusion. It was penetrating every part of my being. When I allowed my mind the freedom to wander, I would find myself deeply saddened. I had to take captive my thoughts and be intentional with my actions.

I had to get up each morning, open the shutters and turn on all the lights, desperate to pierce the darkness. As hard as it was, both physically and emotionally, to get up, get dressed, brush my teeth and wash my face, I had to do it each and every morning.

I owed it to myself, to my family, and to my unborn babies to not let the darkness win. Creating practical steps of action to combat my loneliness would prove a much-needed tool as I learned to navigate the unknown world of mommy-ing multiples.

CHAPTER THREE

The Birth and Recovery

I will not cause pain without allowing something new to be born," says the LORD.

—Isaiah 66:9 NCV

As the weeks crept by, Dr. Browne, Matt, and I had agreed upon a plan of when and how we would deliver the babies. Friday, March 27, would be our scheduled C-section date. We had to find a happy balance between a healthy gestation for the babies and healthy delivery for mommy. The longer they stayed in, the better for them, but the harder for me.

I had been moved back into the hospital as I was having more bouts of preterm labor, and my doctors wanted to keep me closely monitored. I was having trouble internally. As the babies occupied more residence within me, it put pressure on most of my internal organs.

Baby D was so high up that I struggled to breathe, and a kick gone wrong could easily have broken one of my ribs. I was also having extreme burning around my C-section scar, and the doctors feared if I carried on much longer, a uterine rupture was more likely.

All facts considered, we decided on 32 weeks. We had planned for Matt to check the boys out of school early on Thursday and head to Augusta, giving us a chance to enjoy our last afternoon together as a family of four. I don't know why we thought our plan would actually come to fruition when not one of our other plans thus far had. Yet, we were hopeful!

On the morning of March 21, I woke up feeling *off*. I was so groggy I couldn't muster enough energy to eat my breakfast. My nurse thought it was a side effect of the Ambien I was on.

Although I agreed with her, I was confused as to why it had never affected me like that before. I also considered that perhaps I was just sad that Matt and the boys were not coming that weekend since Campbell had a tee-ball game.

I decided to turn off my TV and rest. When the nurse came in later that afternoon and saw uneaten breakfast and lunch trays, my TV off, and me sitting on my bed holding my belly and breathing deeply, she called in the other nurses to get the monitors on me. As they struggled to get the monitors placed, my phone rang. I hadn't spoken to Matt all day and I knew if I didn't answer he would worry.

"Hey, dear," I said shortly.

"Hey honey, You okay? How's your day gone?" he asked.

"Well, not the best. I'm going to need to call you back. They are trying to get these monitors on me and are having a hard time," I explained while trying to shift my large body into a new position.

Once the monitors were in place, I had to lay as still as possible so I would not accidentally bump a monitor out of place. I closed my eyes and tried to rest, but my contractions were becoming more frequent and intense. After 30 minutes of monitoring, the on-call doctor came in.

"Ms. Kirkland, how are you feeling?" he asked, seeming concerned.

I had to fight to catch my breath, "I'm okay."

"How is your pain level?"

"It's pretty high!" I exclaimed. "My scar is really burning and I'm struggling to breathe!"

"I'm going to go call Dr. Browne, but it is my opinion that we should get you prepped for delivery."

"Oh! Tonight? Okay, should I go ahead and call my husband? He is over two hours away."

"Yes ma'am, you should."

After the doctor left the room, I frantically called Matt. Our conversation was short and to the point, as dozens of nurses were continually coming in and out of my room. Within 20 minutes, Dr. Browne had arrived grinning ear to ear.

"So we are doing this tonight then?" he asked excitedly.

"Looks that way," I exhaled.

"Is Matt on his way? Do you want to try and stop labor with magnesium?"

"No!" I shouted, "No! They are ready, I am ready, and Matt is on his way. It's go-time!"

"What about your sister? I know you wanted her here to photograph."

"Unfortunately, she is in Savannah."

"Okay, I can call my daughter. She is a photographer and just happens to be in town visiting."

"I would love that. Thank you."

As Dr. Browne left to call his daughter and prepare for surgery, I called Matt again to see how far away he was. My heart sank when he said he, my mom, and our boys were still an hour away. We quickly had to say our "I love you's," and get off the phone.

The anesthesiologists had just walked in to explain his role in the delivery. Moments after he left, I was wheeled towards the operating room (OR). I was shocked to see 12 NICU nurses lining the hallway, preparing for their roles after delivery.

I smiled, said thank you, and asked each of them to be on their A-game as I passed. Entering the OR, I was even more surprised by the number of people in there. My heart began racing as all 20 of them hustled to set up their delegated work station.

I couldn't believe how many people were required to deliver my babies, and although they were laser-focused, many couldn't help but smile. It was in their smiles that I was reminded of just how extraordinary this delivery would be.

Shortly after receiving my spinal, a nurse approached me and told me my sister Katelyn was there.

"My sister's name is Karen," I said. "I have a cousin named Katelyn."

"Would you like her to come in with you since your husband has yet to arrive?" she asked.

"If she's up for it," I replied.

I lay down on the table as the blue screen went up just below my chest. Katelyn was escorted in moments later to sit on the chair stationed at my head. I asked her to keep talking during the first part and when the babies are about to come, then to stand up and take pictures.

At 7:58 p.m., Ashton Blake Kirkland was born, weighing 3 lbs 6 oz.

A minute later, at 7:59 p.m., Bradlee Ann Kirkland was born, weighing 2 lbs 11 oz.

At 8:00 p.m., Walker Hayes Kirkland arrived, weighing in at 3 lbs 2 oz.

And at 8:02 p.m., Meyers Wayne Kirkland was born, weighing 3 lbs 9 oz.

The moment Dr. Browne called out, "Here comes baby A!" and I heard Ashton's sweet cry, I began to cry. Seeing his tiny, goo-covered body appearing above the blue screen, I cried even more.

Bradlee Ann made herself known as the girl with her high-pitched, squeaky cry. I couldn't believe my girl was finally here. It took five boys to get one girl, and I was elated!

The other two came out like candy from a Pez™ dispenser. Each was rushed to their individual isolette where five nurses awaited them.

I told Katelyn she could leave and show pictures to any family that had arrived. I was praying Matt, the boys, and my mom would arrive in time to see the babies being wheeled out to the NICU.

Unfortunately, they would not make it until much later when I was being wheeled into recovery.

As Katelyn showed my mom and the boys the pictures, Matt ran to be by my side. A wave of peace washed over me the moment I saw his face.

"Good job, Mama! I'm so proud of you!" he said and kissed my forehead.

"I'm so glad you're here! Did you see them?" I asked.

"Not yet. They said it would be at least an hour before anyone can go see them. They have to place their little tubes and monitors."

Although I was so grateful not to be alone in the delivery room, I mourned not being able to share the birth with Matt. I could see in his face he was grateful both the babies and I were okay, but he was devastated he missed their birth.

Luckily, Dr. Browne's daughter was able to tastefully capture every precious moment. Later, all the pictures were put into a slide show so Matt and I were able to experience the birth together in a very special way.

After kissing my sweet boys, I lay in the recovery room exhausted while everyone headed to the cafeteria to get some food. As I closed my eyes, I couldn't help but smile at the miracle I had experienced. I was filled with so much joy, love, and peace. I felt as though God whispered, "Well done!"

✳ ✳ ✳

The Recovery

Growing up an athlete, I was no stranger to injury and the pain associated with it. When I was told having a tubal ligation after the quads were delivered would be painful, I all but laughed the warning off. Man-o-man, I should have heeded that warning!

The gas pains were not normal "gas pains." These gas pains were so severe it felt like my waist was being cinched in two! To make matters worse, I was on a 24-hour IV drip of Pitocin to help shrink my uterus back down to standard postpartum uterus size.

I was in so much pain, it took my husband and a nurse ten minutes to help move me five feet to the bathroom. My legs trembled the whole way, and by the time I reached the bathroom, I was trembling so severely, I couldn't sit down unassisted. Even then, I couldn't relax enough to go pee. I sat on the toilet crying for fifteen minutes before I finally gave up.

I always thought I could do anything. I mean, I just had four babies, but now I couldn't get my body to go pee. Lying back in my bed, I cried even harder knowing that if I was unable to use the bathroom, I would need to have a catheter put back in. Would doing so delay me being able to see my babies?

I was unable to control my emotions. My bladder was full, my waist was being cinched, and I was releasing massive amounts of hormones. Matt did the only thing he knew to do: prayed and then went to get me ice cream.

An hour later, I had to try the bathroom again. I begged for more pain medicine but was denied because morphine had already been added into my spinal before delivery and it lasts up to 24 hours afterward. Oh, DEAR LORD! This was the most excruciating pain I had ever been in, and that was with pain medication!

After two more failed pee attempts, I was finally able to go once we tried a sitz bath. The only one there to celebrate this victory with me was my nurse. Matt and my mom had both gone to go see the babies.

Although I was grateful they were able to go, I couldn't help but be jealous. I desperately wanted my body to hurry and heal enough for me to be able to go to the NICU. I had yet to bond with my babies and the most I had seen of them was from other people's pictures.

I ached to be able to put the tip of my finger into the palm of each little hand and feel their tiny fingers wrap around mine. I feared I was about to battle postpartum depression.

The first time I would be able to see my babies was two agonizing days later, Monday morning at 5:30 a.m. I had been awake for over 36 straight hours, afraid to give in to sleep and miss my opportunity to go to the NICU.

I wanted to see my babies more than I wanted to breathe at this point. I only had to wait for my routine morning blood draw, and then I would be released to go.

As Matt wheeled me into the NICU, my heart raced. I never thought I would have to ask someone which baby was mine.

The uncertainty brought up an uncomfortable level of insecurity within myself. The quads were spread throughout the unit, and the first one we came to was Walker.

"Hey there little guy, Mommy is here! I love you so much!" I whispered between sobs. Just as Matt was about to wheel me to the next baby, a nurse came running to me.

"Your blood results came back with an alarmingly low hemoglobin count. The doctor wants you back downstairs immediately," she exclaimed.

"Can I please just see them all first?" I pleaded. "Even if just for a brief moment?"

"No ma'am, I'm sorry. This is urgent. He wants you back now!" she explained rather harshly.

I looked back at Matt with tears in my eyes, hoping he would fight for me to be able to stay a few more minutes. Instead, I watched the color drain from his face.

"Please? I need to see my babies. They need their mother! They need to know that I'm here." My words were hardly understandable through my sobbing.

"They do need you. So let's get you back downstairs and you can get checked out. The faster we get you well, the faster you can come back to your babies," she said a bit more softly.

Riding the elevator back down, I could see panic consuming my husband. I tried to assure him that I was fine. As the doors opened, we were greeted by two of my nurses waiting to take me back to my room.

They said with my blood level being that low, I shouldn't be able to sit up straight. As soon as we entered the room, my doctor came running in. He took one look at me and looked back down at his paper. "This can't be right," he said. He turned to the nurses and requested another blood draw.

As the nurses rushed the results, Matt sat staring at the floor in a terrified haze.

I tried to comfort him. "Look at me, I am fine! I have color in my face. I am talking and able to sit up. There is no way my blood count is as low as it is showing. I'm no doctor, but on one of my many preterm labor scares, a nurse told me you could not draw blood from the same arm that had the IV of fluids in it. I bet that is why my count is so low," I explained.

I just kept trying to assure him that I was okay, and he just kept staring. Finally, the results came back confirming what I thought had happened. I saw my husband return to normal, so I asked if he would hurry and get me back to the NICU.

Unfortunately, thanks to all the blood draw drama, it was time for the NICU shift change, and it would be another two hours before we would be allowed in.

After a hearty hospital breakfast, Matt once again wheeled me up to the NICU. The pictures did not do my babies justice. They were so tiny. Even through all the machines, tubes, and wires, I was able to see how perfectly God had formed our babies. Each one, unique and beautiful.

Not being able to hold your baby is hard, but having to ask permission to put your hand through their isolette required a whole different level of strength, one that no mother should have to endure. As much as I hated it, I followed all the rules. I would deny my challenger nature to be able to see and touch my babies.

Three short days after I gave birth to four babies, I was being discharged from the hospital. No one could believe it. Our insurance company wouldn't even cover one day per baby? Not to mention I still couldn't walk!

Just the day before, I was in so much pain I had to be given a morphine shot in my leg in order to function enough to get into my wheelchair to go see the babies. Nevertheless, I was being released, so I did what any desperate mother would do. I stole a wheelchair.

Over the next four days, I would wheel myself from the RMH to the NICU, and no one was any the wiser. Once I was able to walk again, I wheeled myself into the hospital elevator, and once I reached the NICU floor, I walked myself out!

CHAPTER FOUR

Close the Window

We can make our plans,
but the LORD determines our steps.

—Proverbs 16:9 NLT

B eing pregnant with high order multiples, super twins, grand multiples, whichever name you prefer, is not easy. Being pregnant is not easy. At least it never was for me. But carrying four babies at one time kicked up the intensity level a notch ... or four!

All symptoms (nausea, fatigue, heartburn, itchy palms, hemorrhoids) and baby movements (hiccups, flutters, kicks, turnovers) were exaggerated. I could no longer rely on my experience with my other two kids because this pregnancy was a whole new ball game.

* * *

To this day Matt and I catch ourselves smiling and nodding when we hear other parents complaining about how hard they have it with their little one. Don't get me wrong, each pregnancy and each child is unique, and we should save ourselves the pain of comparing our situation to someone else's.

The truth is, another family's struggle is truth for them and is justified for them; nonetheless, we smile. I like to use the analogy of high school level sports versus college-level sports. Both have their own unique challenges, but college sports are played at a higher level of intensity.

* * *

Every time I formed a plan based on my previous experience, my plan went right out the window. I planned to visit and tour both hospitals in our town to be able to make an educated decision on which hospital I felt would be the best fit for me and our babies. Nope, that plan went out the window when the hospital I would deliver at was decided for me.

I planned to have the nursery put together in beautiful coordinating layettes before I went on bed rest. Nope! Our budget, or lack thereof, threw that plan out the window.

Out of an eight-piece nursery set (times four), I was able to get the one set of the curtains I wanted. I planned for 32 pieces total, and I got two! And they didn't arrive until after I had been sent away.

Typically, moms experience a nesting phase where they feel a deep-rooted desire to organize and prepare for their baby. I enjoyed nesting with my other two. It helped me to feel accomplished in knowing that when the baby was born, he would return to a nursery that was properly organized.

Clothes were washed and hung by size, diapers out of the packaging and placed evenly on the changing table alongside the stocked wipes, baby lotion, and pee-pee teepees (cone-shaped pieces of fabric, that are placed on your baby boy's sprayer while changing his diaper).

Blankets would be folded on their proper shelf in the closet beside the folded receiving blankets, not to be confused with the light-weight linen swaddle blankets that hung separately.

Stuffed animals were arranged so only the softest was placed in the far corner of the crib. The rest were placed in various locations in small clusters to give the illusion that a particular spot was a loving, welcoming, and friendly location.

Seems silly, but when I was nesting, it seemed necessary. I love a well-thought-out and executed plan, and I was constantly being disappointed that my quad plans were not going according to plan.

Every week at my doctor's appointment, we would set a plan based on my current condition. And every week our plan changed. Despite my efforts, my conditions and circumstances were *always* changing.

As frustrated and discouraged as the changes left me feeling, I learned a valuable life lesson. Never base a plan on your current conditions and circumstances because they are always changing! Not just for moms of multiples, for everyone. There is a universal law called the Law of Vibration. This law simply states that all things are in a constant state of movement.

Movement, whether I like it or not, equals change. There is no emotional pain that comes from change; pain comes from the fear of change. The pain comes from staying still while everything around you continues to move.

I fought this notion of movement because I was on bed rest. My ability to move was restricted. If only universal laws worked that way. But, alas, they do not. That's why they are universal, they apply to everyone and don't discriminate by life's circumstance.

* * *

When I was away, I did my best to stay actively involved with my company back home. I would Skype in for staff meetings, talk to managers and my partner almost daily. And for the first few weeks, I would log in remotely to do payroll.

*When I do payroll, I like to put a little inspirational quote in the memo line. As I was skimming through the material of John Maxwell (the number one leadership expert in the world who would later become my mentor) because he has some great one-liners, I stopped and decided to start from the beginning of my **21 Irrefutable Laws of Leadership**[1] book. I had the time. Why not?*

The name of the first law mentioned is "The Law of the Lid." Within moments of skimming, I was bawling! The law simply means that a company, organization, or what have you, can only grow to the level of its leader!

If I am an average leader (a level 5), my company can never grow beyond a level 4.

Light bulbs were exploding everywhere! (No, not literally!) This "AHA" moment was gargantuan to me. I had been feeling such pressure, and not just from inside my uterus, but from everywhere. My company was growing rapidly and my family was about to double. I had to personally grow so that everything else could grow.

* * *

I may not be able to change my conditions and circumstances; however, I can grow my level of awareness in how I operate within them. One of my favorite quotes is: "Set a goal so big that you can't achieve it until you grow into the person who can!"

I knew from the moment of hearing that fourth heart beat that God's plan was far greater than any plan I could have ever imagined for myself. I also knew I could not work in his plan without him and the people he would place in my life to help me.

As I mentioned before, I love a well-thought-out and executed plan. The challenge I face with working in God's plan is that you have to suspend knowing the answer to *how?* **Working in God's plan calls for steps of faith, not steps of certainty.**

In carrying four babies, having my other two boys and husband at home, and running a company, I yearned for steps of certainty. I wanted to know when these babies would be born. I wanted to know how long they would be in the NICU. I wanted to know when we would be allowed to go back home. I wanted to know if and when they would sleep through the night.

I wanted to know how my company would continue to grow in my absence. I wanted to know how my husband's business partners would support whatever choices he had to make in order to have more time with his sons and time to visit his wife ... and have time to spend with his babies once they did come home!

I wanted—I needed—certainty in all those things, plus many more. But God was calling me to faith by obedience. To bring my burdens and troubled heart to him, not because of what I would get in doing so, but in who he was molding me to be.

Decisions of obedience are easy when you know the outcome. I would pray for the answer to the how. Oftentimes, I was asked: *How are you going to be able to run a company and have six kids? How are you going to feed four babies? There's no way to do it all, you will have to sell your company! How in the world would you be able to afford childcare for four babies? You know you will need lots of help—how are you going to get the help you need?*

How are you going to _____? (fill in the blank).

I was surrounded by people's genuine curiosity in *how* I was going to make it all work. I would smile and give my best guess, or I would say, "I don't know." And that was the truth.

All my previous plans had gone out the window, so I was hesitant to plan for anything anymore. I had grown bitter towards planning. In hindsight, I know that there is, absolutely, a place for planning.

In fact, another favorite quote I often use in my company is: "Failing to plan is planning to fail." There is truth in that statement, and as much as I love it, I have amended it to the following: "Failing to plan is planning to fail; however, if the plan fails, allow yourself the grace to accept it and hold tight to your vision and the 'why' that created it to keep you moving forward."

When I was on bedrest, someone asked me *how* I was going to do something, and I made my best-educated guess on the subject. I wish I had the foresight to tell her, "I don't know *how* I'm going to do it ... but after I've done it, I'll tell you *how* I did it."

Now, being able to operate at this higher level of awareness brings greater peace to my life. I don't have to know all—or any—of the answers. Believe me, I still LOVE to have the answers, but in the field of mommy-ing multiples plus two, being a wife, and running a company, I have accepted the truth that a step in obedient faith is far more rewarding than a step of what the world offers as certainty.

I still plan, but I also plan for failure, because failure is only failure when you quit and have learned nothing. You can have all the experiences, but they will never be as good as evaluated experiences.

So when I fail, I only allow myself a brief moment of pity. The "Oh, woe is me" time has its rightful place. But I keep the moment to that ... a moment.

One of my favorite sayings in times of sadness is "This too shall pass." The reality is, this statement is true for good times as well. No time, be it good or bad, lasts. My goal is to give thanks for and enjoy the good and to learn and grow from the bad.

In not being able to close the window my plans are always flying out of, I have learned to jump out with them, creating my wings to fly on the way down. I don't often know how I'm going to accomplish a goal until I have done it. Thanks to having quadruplets, I know I am far more capable than I ever imagined possible. But in the moments of feeling "Super Mom" status ... I was quickly humbled.

CHAPTER FIVE

Celebrity

For we walk by faith, not by sight.

—2 Corinthians 5:2 KJ21®

I have yet to meet someone—especially a woman—who enjoys being humbled. Possibly ... looong after the act, sure ... but during? As I said, I have yet to meet someone. I don't mind being wrong. Of course, I prefer to be right; however, if I err, I take responsibility for it. I don't have to *be* right—I have to get it right!

I had moments of feeling I deserved the title of SuperMom! I remember the first day I was alone with all four babies. They were eating every three hours, and with each feeding I alternated which baby I would nurse, while the other three received a propped bottle.

* * *

Side note on bottle propping: This subject is a hot-button topic for many parents. Matt and I were aware of the safety risks of leaving a baby propped to eat by himself. Never once were our babies left unsupervised while being propped.

We would arrange three babies, tilted slightly on their sides, on my pregnancy body pillow, or they would have their own individual Boppy™. We then would place a burp cloth between their little chins and the Zakys™ (best purchase ever) we used to hold the bottle.

A Zaky is made specifically as a positioner for babies. Moms and Dads sleep with the Zaky, allowing the material to absorb their scent. The Zaky (shaped like a hand and forearm) is placed in the bassinet, or incubator with the baby. Once our babies were out of the NICU, the Zakys made great bottle props.

* * *

For my first solo feeding, I prepared the bottles, gathered my supplies (bibs, burp cloths, Zakys, Boppies), and set up the floor with three babies creating a semi-circle in front of me while I nursed the other. Twenty-eight minutes later, all babies were fed, burped, changed, swaddled, and laid back to sleep.

I wanted a pat on the back. I wanted to toot my own horn. I did a little dance of joy and then, like much of my journey, I filmed the whole feeding and posted it to the Quads Facebook page. I got the props I was searching for ... and I felt great.

Before the babies were born, and I had been moved away to Augusta, I was on modified bed rest at home. I did a lot of Googling on quads, quad births, quad pregnancies ... you name it, I searched it.

On one of my searches, I stumbled upon a Facebook page of a fellow quad mom whose birth announcement had gone viral. She had just had her babies, and they were all doing well. I posted a note of congratulations and told her I was 20-weeks pregnant with quads and thanked her for sharing her journey.

I got off my computer and went about the rest of my day.

Everything seemed ... no, "seemed" is too generous ... every-thing was *hard! Feeding, diapering, sleeping ... not sleeping, big kids, being a wife, laundry ... oh so much laundry, self-care ... or lack thereof, and that was just at home.*

While still in the RMH, I signed up to join the John Maxwell Team, after I had the realization that I needed to "lift my lid," meaning I had to grow to a higher level of leadership so that my company could reach a higher level.

I enrolled and began studying. It was easy while I was alone and on bed rest to read, reflect, journal, and take courses; but now that we were all back home, desperately trying to make it hour by hour, my personal growth plan was reduced and put on the back burner to simmer.

Yet, I still had a business to run, I still had a team that counted on me, and truth-be-told, I still needed and wanted to work.

Mom-ing is, in my opinion, the hardest and most rewarding job (not financially, cause you don't get paid to mommy ... cause no one could afford you ... just sayin')! I was called to work outside the home as well.

I have so much passion for adding value to people, loving and leading others as Jesus so freely does for me, and providing a safe environment for people to grow—in an environment that encourages fresh starts and new hope.

My company was and is my ministry. To be able to carry out my company vision, I still had to be involved; we had yet to grow to having multiple shareholders who would carry out the vision in my absence.

At this particular moment, that responsibility rested on my shoulders. My business was growing rapidly and I had begun to entertain the idea of expanding to multiple locations. (I know ... even writing this I'm thinking how crazy I was.)

My entrepreneurial drive heated up and my simmering pot began to boil!

* * *

Rapidly growing in all areas of life caused my focus and time to shift. Every moment was used up.

Creating new content for my blog and Facebook page was no longer something I enjoyed; it began to feel like an obligation. I had grown so fond of my followers and really enjoyed the connections I had made, yet I simply had no time. And I am a huge proponent of making time for what's important, but, at the end of the day, sharing my life was nowhere near as important as trying to survive it!

I minimally updated my page with pictures and anecdotes a few times a month to appease those who had come to care for me and my babies. I only shared in my integrity of wanting to, not the notion that I had to, or that I owed it to anyone.

I was and will always be grateful for their support and encouragement during one of the hardest times in my life. Even though my social media presence was lacking, we still had newspapers, magazines, and TV producers wanting to share our story.

Atlanta magazine wanted to do a feature on us and would send a photographer out several times over the course of several months in order to best capture our reality. After setting some ground rules (i.e. gently sharing my trepidation caused by the troll experience), we agreed to the magazine. Both the writer and photographer were kind and creative, resulting in a beautifully composed feature.

A week after the magazine published, I received a Facebook message from a TV producer's assistant. I was skeptical, but after doing my due diligence, I discovered all was legit. The producer went back and forth for almost a year with TLC, UP, and a few other networks trying to get a deal.

We were not willing to do *reality for ratings;* we wanted our show to be an accurate depiction of our lives. Unfortunately (in some aspects) and fortunately (in many aspects), a deal was never reached and we carried on with our happy, chaotic lives.

When we were first in talks with the production company, I remember Matt and I talking and praying together, wondering if this is why God gave us six kids.

Matt had only ever wanted one child, and I have never considered myself a good mothering type. We were not sitting pretty financially. We thought maybe TV was meant to be our platform to share our story, our love, and our faith with others.

We thought a show would be how we were able to provide for our family financially. (I mean, how else does one afford six kids?) At the very least, we thought having a show would provide us with professional recordings of our family to cherish forever.

At this moment in time, we were well aware of my dad's Alzheimer's, and I thought, just maybe, TV was God's plan to open new doors of opportunity to be able to get my dad more help. Perhaps it would bring awareness to the struggles both the family and the patient face with this horrible disease.

I thought I would have my kids growing up on film, so if I were ever to be diagnosed, I would have my memories recorded for me.

Fortunately, God's provision allowed for our family to grow and go through our trials, tribulations, and loss away from the public eye and the scrutiny that comes with it.

Having been through the troll experience previously, we handled the rejection well.

CHAPTER SIX

The Illusion

As water reflects the face, so one's life reflects the heart.

—Proverbs 27:19 NIV

Despite the kind, supportive words from all those who had been following our journey, calling me Super Mom, Wonder Woman, Rock Star, etc., I was anything but. Although the encouragement was nice to hear, and often an appreciated boost in my confidence, the truth was our journey was hard.

Many days I would pray for the strength to make it to the next minute, not day, not week—but minute! I didn't want to give any illusions that I actually knew what I was doing or that I had anything figured out.

In blogging, I had always promised raw honesty. I felt it was extremely important for anyone who was reading to know that I was not so good at sugar-coating. I tell it like it is ... no illusions.

When I was pregnant, I was under so many illusions from other moms of multiples who seemed to take their journey so much easier ... pools or hydrotherapy tubs to help soothe their achy bodies, C-sections that seemed to be no big deal, recoveries that appeared to be mess-free in their silk pajamas, NICU suites, and policies that appeared to not demand a yellow gown cover for sanitary purposes, or that let the parents hold their babies whenever.

I gazed in wonder at photos of postpartum bodies that were tight and back to prepregnancy weight within a few weeks. All illusions! All the aforementioned scenarios were not even *close* to my experience.

Every time I hit a new step in my journey, I made the mistake of comparing it to someone else's and when my scenario did not replicate hers, I found myself disappointed.

Why were my stepping stones always boulders?

So in my blog, I wanted to clear the air and give hope to anyone who had not had it easy. Sometimes life hands you a lemon and when you go to make lemonade, you are out of sugar.

I was not about to pretend I could do this mommy-ing multiples thing on my own, using my own strength. I had no more strength. It was amazing how quickly lack of sleep depleted my strength.

I knew that without the Lord, I would crumble into an emotional mess. He kept me functioning when I felt I could function no more. He had shown me grace and mercy that sustained and revived me.

In the day-to-day, I was beyond thankful for the support of my family, my babysitter, and the countless people who had offered support with meals, diapers, wipes, letters of encouragement, extra hands around the house, and arms to hold babies.

* * *

There was one afternoon in particular that will be forever treasured. Swaying while looking out my dining room window, impatiently awaiting the desperately needed help, I saw Matt's aunts and uncle unloading a car full of diapers, wipes, and food to stock our freezer.

I was so overcome with gratitude, I almost dropped the two babies I was soothing to rush outside to welcome them. They stayed with us for a week, cooking, cleaning, and generally being helpful.

They instinctively did everything I didn't even know I needed. Sitting up late one night talking to Matt's aunts while they helped me feed the babies, I began to get emotional.

Matt had lost his dad suddenly the year we married and, eight years later, his dad's sisters would be sitting with me reminiscing beautiful stories of a father-in-law I never got to know.

Through them, our children would acquire bonus grand-parents.

Through them, I would get to experience the love and support Matt's father would have offered.

Through them, I could see Matt's father, sitting in his old wooden rocking chair, eyes beaming through his large-framed glasses, cradling a baby ever so tenderly.

He would be quietly humming his favorite hymns, only stopping to softly kiss the sweet forehead of his baby's beautiful baby while whispering an "I love you."

He would look up, grinning cheek to cheek, to tell his only son how proud of him he was.

I never would have anticipated the depth of the connection I would feel to Matt's father through his aunts.

* * *

Before the babies were even born, I was grateful for my mom and sister going above and beyond to make sure Campbell and Jack's world kept spinning while mine seemed to be standing still.

I was grateful for my aunt who taught me how to knit soft, little blankets for each baby. She would drive down to Augusta, knit and chat with me about my cousin's upcoming wedding, helping take me out of my own head and be excited for others.

I cannot find the words to express how thankful I am for all those who so generously loved on our family when we needed it most. I cannot fathom how difficult life would have been without all the support we received.

As the quads grew, so did my fear of not being good enough. I was already struggling with mom-ing six, though four of them were still under constant care by the nurses at the NICU. I knew deep in my heart that God was still in control; however, my mind would often drift into a sea of doubt.

My babies were only 37-weeks gestation at six weeks old. They were preemies and pretty much slept until it was time to wake and eat, then it was right back to sleep. I looked forward to, yet still feared, the newborn stage.

They would be awake more often and be in need of entertaining! *That was a full-time job with one baby—how could a mom do it with four?* I was fortunate early on that my babies were tiny enough that I could scoop up one with one arm while still holding another. *But how in the world could I do that once they started getting bigger and gaining weight?* I was no Super Woman.

As all the hours ran together, I often had to backtrack two or three feedings to recall a start time, then I would just add the necessary three hours between feedings to get to the start time I was seeking. I made many mistakes and was often in a state of exhaustion and confusion.

I had fed the same baby twice. In the middle of the night, I had forgotten to feed the baby that was lying on top of my chest. I had told the hubs I would breastfeed her, and then we both passed out!

I had gone until 2 p.m. without a bite to eat ... and those who know me know how *huge* that was. (I like to eat lunch at 10:45 a.m.)

I had learned that I could carry on a full conversation with my husband while I was completely asleep.

I constantly smelled of spit up since two of the four had terrible reflux. It was amazing how I could come out of the shower still smelling of spit up! But I was thankful for the shower, nonetheless, because those were few and far between.

Even during the day, I was constantly falling asleep while breastfeeding. Thankfully, Jack or Campbell would yell at me to wake up, and thankfully I was always in a safe place with a big Boppy pillow around me.

I loathed cleaning bottles—unscrewing all the various parts, making sure every crevice was cleaned completely; otherwise, the next time I went to make a bottle, I would gag at the putrid odor that lingered.

I would gladly change diapers in lieu of cleaning bottles. It was the worst part of my day. I was greeted every morning with the kitchen sink full of all the prior night's bottles. There was no avoiding it—the sink was right beside the coffee pot!

I was astonished that even with breastfeeding, we were going through a can of formula every two days. I fervently prayed that God would maintain my milk supply and allow it to grow as the babies did.

Every drop of milk produced was coveted. Not just for the benefits of breastmilk and the money it saved, but it meant fewer bottles to have to wash!

With all the burp cloths, bibs, Boppy covers, soiled cloth diapers, and spit up-saturated onesies, we ended up getting a second washer and dryer.

Through it all, Matt and I still couldn't believe we had been asked to reduce. We were so blessed by all of our children, even though we got no sleep and I had developed an eye twitch caused by exhaustion.

One of my favorite moments happened when I was breastfeeding two babies; Matt was bottle feeding one and burping another, and he looked at each baby for a moment then looked at me and said, "Reduce? My ass!"

Funny? Yes! But it was so precious to me because when we were talking of having a second child, Matt's biggest concern was that he wouldn't have enough love for another baby. And there we were, years later with six kids.

Our hearts were overflowing with so much love that we couldn't imagine life without each one of them.

To this day, when I look at my six healthy and happy miracles, I am able to see how their lives reflect their hearts ...

With Campbell, a.k.a. "Bubs," I am blessed by his obedient nature and kind heart. I can always count on him to help.

With Jack, a.k.a. "Doodle Bug," I am always laughing! His zeal for creativity entertains us all.

With Ashton, a.k.a. "The Big Guy" (as he stands a head above the others), I am amazed at how his loving and responsible character is positioning him as the leader of the four.

With Bradlee, a.k.a. "Girl" (because not only is she the only girl, but she is also a girly girl), I am grateful for how her gentle and kind spirit calms the 100-mph speed at which our house typically functions. God knew the exact girl we needed to handle a house full of boys!

With Walker, a.k.a. "Walkie," I am enthralled by his creative zest for life and curiosity for discovery. He keeps us on our toes.

With Meyers, a.k.a. "Meyerszaz," I am reminded of the importance of imagination and how our minds are our greatest resource. Meyers' ability to create is inspiring.

Because having six kids is like being hooked up to an IV of humility, I am grateful to remain grounded without any illusions. Choosing to see the beauty in our chaos at times may be hard, but the joy it brings to my heart is worth it.

For as he thinketh in his heart, so is he.

—Proverbs 23:7 (KJV)

CHAPTER SEVEN

Beauty and the Believer

God is within her, she will not fail.

—Psalm 46:5 NIV

I dreamed of being a dolphin trainer when I grew up. There was a brief period when I thought I wanted to be in the medical field, but that was more for secure income than living out any passion or purpose. I never once, not one single time, thought I would grow up and run a salon company. Not ever. Not … one … time.

Nevertheless, I found myself working the front desk for a salon one spring, no magical connection, no divine calling. I simply was working a job that I didn't hate, and that I didn't come home from smelling like food!

There were a few times I wanted to quit, to figure out my passion, but I heard how much fun the company Christmas parties were, so I stuck around. After all, I had my priorities. That first company Christmas party was not as epic as it was made out to be, but whenever I felt the urge to look elsewhere for employment opportunities, I hung on. I was engaged and I really didn't want to have to pay full price for my wedding hair (insert facepalm emoji here)!

I cringe looking back at that time of my life. I had no idea about anything. I was just living a surface-level life and was none the wiser to it. It wouldn't be until after Campbell was born that my life would get a whole lot deeper.

I stayed on with the salon company after Matt and I got married, not for a Christmas party, not for more of my hair needs, but because I had formed a genuine love for the people and the work I was doing. I wasn't doing the hair. I was growing the people and the business. As I did so, my passion for adding value to others began to take root.

I would continue on with this salon company through my first child and halfway through the pregnancy of my second. When I was six months pregnant with Jack, Matt and I decided that I should stay home.

I loved being with Campbell (our firstborn, who was now one and a half). We would be able to save money not having to pay for childcare. I was sure I would be the *best* stay-at-home mom. The house would be clean, the homemade dinners served. We would do crafts and sing songs. Heck, I might even homeschool!

By the time Jack was six months old, I was desperate to get back into the salon. Being a stay-at-home mom was the hardest job ever. I loved being with my kids, but I quickly learned I am a much better mommy when I am not with my kids 24/7.

I had tried getting my old job back, but the replacement I trained was doing well and all they could offer me was a part-time front desk shift (the same shift, with the same pay I had started with over five years earlier).

I did not dismiss the offer, but I had to seriously pray about it. If I would be spending time away from my children, it had to be worth it. If not financially, then it had to serve my passion.

I am an entrepreneur down to every cell in my body, although I would not understand that about myself until several years later. I had always been competitive with others and with myself. I didn't give up easily; I was always driven to either find a way or make a way. I knew I was being called to more.

Growing up, I had asked Jesus into my heart when I was very young, and although I talked to God daily, I didn't fully understand what living for Christ meant.

Later in high school, on September 11, 2001, after watching the terrorist attack on our nation on the TV in our math class, I came home from school deeply grieved. I remember watching the news coverage as I sat on the arm of our living room couch with tears streaming down my face.

I prayed for God's peace, for understanding, for our nation, and that God would use me for good as I walked in obedience to him.

Years went by and my faith neither grew nor left me. I was just living my life. That was, until I had Campbell. The moment I held him, I knew I could and would lay down my life for him. The nurse came in to take him to get cleaned up, and I remember thinking, *"If she hurts my baby, I will end her."* Dramatic, I know, but I had so many hormones racing through me.

Again that evening, holding my precious and clean baby I understood. I understood the enormity of the sacrifice of Jesus. I prayed, *"Lord, thank you for loving me! If you can die for me, then I can live for you."*

I believe God had always been with me, waiting, available, willing to show himself whenever I was willing to see him. The turning point in my faith journey happened the night Campbell was born. I shifted from living my life for me, seeing God only when times were really good or really bad, to living my life for him, seeing God in everything! My passion for adding value to people had taken root, but now my purpose was beginning to bud.

Here I was, a mom of two young boys, wanting to get back into the workforce, and show an industry—which, on a surface level, is based on vanity—the love, compassion, and hope that Christ had shown me. Sorella Hair Studio would be a place for women to love, support, and encourage one another—like family! After all, Sorella is Italian for "sister."

I was 29 years old, being called to open my own salon without a college degree. I never doubted my ability to run a business. I did, however, doubt if the banks would have as much confidence in me as I had in myself.

Matt agreed I could go for it, with the understanding that I was not allowed to offer our home as collateral, he could not co-sign with me, or be attached to my company since that could impact his company.

I was so naive about what to ask for from the bank. Everything I knew about creating a business plan came from Google. Nevertheless, I composed my general business plan and went to the bank:

Hi, I have been a stay at home mom for a year and a half. I have no money and no form of collateral. I have never owned a business, and I would like to open my own salon company. Will you give me money to do so?

Rightly so, the bank rejected me.

I was devastated.

I felt so defeated. Why would they not loan me the money? Salons make money, I had salon experience, I was getting into it for the right reasons, I mean … I had a business plan! Had I misunderstood what God was calling me to do?

mon area maintenance) would increase, along with the number of repairs and amount of maintenance that we incurred on taking over an older space. Every spring and summer, our air conditioning would go out.

We were doing so much business that we had to have another water heater installed just to be able to keep up. The water heater expense was one that couldn't wait long because by 2 p.m. every day, we were out of hot water!

"So sorry for the cold plunge you are about to receive. The good part is, rinsing your hair in cold water helps lock in your color."

Money needed to open a business is different from money needed to run a business—a lesson I wish I had learned on someone else's dime.

Coming into our third year, we were simply breaking even. Even with month after month of watching our sales increase, the excitement was short-lived as, in order to reach our profit numbers, we needed to be doing $20K more a month!

Even using all my creative entrepreneurial tactics, such as leveraging services in exchange for marketing, using any and all forms of free social media marketing, etc., there was no physical way to increase our guest count enough without more stylists to do the hair.

We couldn't add more stylists without adding more stations. We couldn't add more stations without investing more money into renovations. And on top of it all, I was now pregnant with quadruplets!

Listening to everyone else, including the doctors, telling me that there was no way I would be able to carry these babies, no way I could run a business and a house of six kids, no way my marriage would be strong enough, there would be no way (fill in the blank) ... I almost believed them.

But one of my favorite things about me is *my desire to persevere.* I am not afraid to take on a challenge. In fact, I thrive on it. I love finding ways to make things work, to figure out the solutions. I had never been a quitter and wasn't about to start now. I knew that whenever I was at my weakest, God would come through in a mighty way, giving me the strength to keep moving forward.

"Let me tell you something you already know. The world ain't all sunshine and rainbows. It's a very mean and nasty place and I don't care how tough you are, it will beat you to your knees and keep you there permanently if you let it. You, me, or nobody is gonna hit as hard as life. But it ain't about how hard ya hit. It's about how hard you can get hit and keep moving forward. How much you can take and keep moving forward. That's how winning is done!" —Rocky Balboa.²

I used to watch the *Rocky* movies with my dad, just to spend time with him. I didn't care much for the movies, but I would watch anything to spend a few hours with him, and in doing so, that quote would imbed itself in my mind for many years to come.

Never underestimate a mama who's got God within her and a good *Rocky* quote in her back pocket!

By the time the quads were one, I was preparing to open a second salon location. This new location would be almost quadruple the size of my original location. (Hello, God wink … look at that math!)

I would not only be running another commissioned salon within it but I would also be building out separate salon suites within the space to allow for rental income.

I knew not everyone was destined to be a commissioned employee. I knew there was a place for it. And I also knew there was a need for rental space.

There were several booth/station rent salons in our town, but I wanted to create separate suites. The suites would offer an independent stylist the opportunity to run her own salon, without all the overhead, making it more profitable than a traditional salon.

This new business model would allow me to reach and add value to even more people, which aligned with my passion.

Still carrying debt from our original location, I knew I would not be able to do another SBA loan. I also knew that this time I would have to offer up some collateral to be able to secure financing.

This time I was certain I would ask for enough money to not only build out the space we needed but also to be able to open and *run* the business ... unlike my previous experience. I was also holding onto the idea of merging the two salons together in a little over a year when I would have the opportunity to not renew my current lease with Publix. I would once again be able to secure a loan, but this time, our house would be on the line.

CHAPTER EIGHT

A Crappy Situation

He calms the storm and stills the waves.

—Psalm 107:29 TLB

For the next year, I would continue to run both salon locations while running a home with two-year-old quadruplets, a six-year-old, an eight-year-old, two dogs, a cat, and a husband.

Life was about to show up!

Having two-year-old quadruplets is, to date, one of the hardest things I have had to endure. The unspeakable chaos and destruction the quads caused earned them the moniker QUADNADO (think tornado, but with kids ... and more destructive!) Still, I think the hardest part was the constant navigating of unknown territory.

* * *

Challenges in life are always met with more difficulty when you don't know what to expect, but then again, isn't that what makes life challenging? Not knowing what to expect—the fear of the unknown—can be debilitating for many.

Many dear friends suffer from clinical anxiety, which is more than just sweaty palms, accelerated pulse, and feeling nervous.

I once saw a meme that classified anxiety symptoms as follows:

1. Never sitting down to relax

2. Always checking phone

3. Overachiever—type A personality

4. Never able to switch off from work

5. Quick to judge/criticize others

6. Zoning out of conversations

7. Angry outbursts at loved ones

8. Avoiding social situations

9. Sweaty palms

10. Excessive drinking of alcohol

11. Binge-eating junk foods

12. Watching hours of television

13. Online shopping addiction

Although I understand the awareness this meme is trying to bring about, I was struck with concern.

Knowing people who greatly suffer with anxiety, memes like this, seen out of context, can give someone the excuse of crying "anxiety" when that might not truly be the case.

Stress, anxiety, and depression are serious and should be taken as such. Sadly, at least in my experience with the salon industry, I am seeing that the more creative a person is, the more these mental stressors tend to plague her.

I have tightly held the shoulders of one of my employees who was physically shaking, rocking, sweating, and crying during an anxiety attack.

I may have anxious thoughts and feelings, but I am able to mentally get myself out of it.

I know that physiologically speaking, my body does not know the difference between an excited emotion and an anxious emotion, as both involve butterflies, sweaty palms, accelerated heart rate, and nervous feelings, so I am able to use my mental faculties to navigate my way through anxious moments. For me to claim to have anxiety would be desensitizing the severity of one who truly suffers from this form of mental illness.

One of the most extreme cases of anxiety I have personally known was with my sister-in-law. Matt called me one Friday afternoon saying his sister was suffering extreme panic attacks and he needed to fly to Kansas to rent a car and drive her back to Georgia.

My husband is by no means a "fly by the seat of your pants" kind of guy. He likes to figure things out. He takes time to process and research all the ins and outs! So when he told me he was en route to the airport, I knew it was serious.

Matt has never really understood much about mental illness and even had some judgments about it. I think many of our judgments about others stem from our own insecurity and lack of understanding.

His sister's severe anxiety prevented them from being able to board a plane and fly back to Georgia. He would spend the next few days driving many miles, experiencing a whole new level of understanding about what anxiety can do to someone.

It was a horrible experience for both Matt and his sister to have to endure, but they did it together! Matt learned that even if you don't fully understand why and how something is happening, you can still have compassion for those who are going through it.

After my miscarriage and again after my dad died, I would go through a rough time working through depression; however, I will not claim to have been depressed.

*The words we speak are extremely powerful! We not only say them ... we hear them, causing a higher degree of penetration into our subconscious mind. Working through depression is an effort I took on; whereas, claiming to **be depressed** would be depression taking over me, giving more power to the action.*

One who truly suffers from diagnosed chronic mental illness may not have the same abilities to get themselves out of it the way someone who is in a season of mental distress.

Don't hear what I'm not saying. When you are in it ... it is awful, be it chronic or short-lived, it's awful! The dark cloud of sorrow that seems to be consuming your light, the unseen weight that crushes your chest is real and needs to be addressed appropriately.

✳ ✳ ✳

Being a parent for the first time can be filled with anxious moments. Being a parent to preemie quadruplets definitely was! I felt much more comfortable about my abilities as a mom than I was with newborn Campbell.

With my first baby, I would walk to the edge of my stairs and call Matt to tell him I was about to carry our baby downstairs. If he didn't get a call from me in the next minute, he needed to call 911. I was beyond terrified and felt completely inadequate in caring for our new baby. Thankfully, as I imagine it is with most new moms, I learned quickly.

After having two kids, I had developed some mad mommy skills; however, I was crazy unprepared for the whole new, elevated level of parenting that quadruplets required.

In most cases, a mom can go pick up her crying child to comfort her when needed, or allow her to fall asleep cuddled gently in the crook of her arm. This experience was something I took for granted with both of my singletons.

When all four babies are crying at the same time, you don't have enough crooks in which to comfort. I would make sure they were safe in their cribs and then would walk downstairs, sit in my recliner with a bowl of ice cream, rocking and crying because I could not hold and comfort all four of my babies at once.

If one cried more severely than the rest, I would sneak into their room, crawling on the floor to the individual's crib, grab the baby, and strategically inchworm my way back out of the room. Downstairs, I rocked and comforted that baby alone. As the babies grew, they became little pros at self-soothing, so when one would outcry the others, the rest would settle themselves, knowing that their sibling needed care.

They developed their own way of communicating with each other early in life. It was a cool phenomenon to experience!

What was not cool was when the quads were two and they

went through a poop art phase. This phase, although comical to the outsider, beat me down like no other has ... thus far ... in my current ten years of parenting.

We tried everything to curtail the poop: clothes on backward, duct tape, cloth diapers, disposable diapers ... You name it, we tried it! But despite our exhaustive and best efforts, the poop prevailed.

I could not leave the room without returning to a poo-nami! I would even wait for all four to poop before I would lay them down for their nap, yet ... somehow, one, two, three, or all four mustered up some poop to create—in their minds—beautiful works of poop art.

Matt and I still laugh (now, not then—we cried then!) about the time he came home from work and went in their room to play with them while I fixed dinner. About 10 minutes later, he headed to the big boys' room to chat with them about their day.

Shortly after that, I heard a loud, oddly high-pitched, man-scream echo through the house. He had walked back into the babies' room only to meet fresh poop art!

"NOOOO! **WHY?** *Why do you guys always have to poop and play with it? I haven't even been gone for five minutes! How is this even possible! That's it, Julie ... our kids are going to be the end of me! We should not have to live in* **FEAR**, *that every time we walk out of the room, we are going to come back to* **POOP EVERYWHERE!**"

Now my husband has a pretty deep voice, but when he intensely screams, he can get as squeaky as a preteen boy entering puberty!

As trying, gross, and exhausting as the poo phase was, it wasn't the only crap I was having to deal with. My two salon companies had managed to build up resentment towards each other.

I was bouncing back and forth between both locations for only a few hours a day (because paying for full-time child care for quadruplets was more per month than our mortgage, so we settled for help three to four hours a day, three days per week).

Thus, the time I was able to be in each individual salon and work with my team was short-lived.

One of the best parts about owning a business is having the freedom to set your own schedule. One of the hardest parts about owning a business that involves growing, developing, and investing in people, is they want you around to do so.

I was not only seeing jealousy forming at home over where my attention went, but now also at work. Yet these were grown adults!

I was doing my best and it simply was not good enough.

Why did I have to be so ambitious? Why did I bite off more than I could chew … or even put in my mouth? Why did no one seem to care that I was trying? Why did I keep overpromising and under-delivering? Why was "work/life balance" proving to be impossible? Why was it all so hard?

Our locations were on opposite sides of town, so we referred to them as Eastside and Westside … big mistake! Like I have mentioned before, I believe in the power of our words and nicknaming our salons would just add fuel to the fire of the *Westside Story* vibes we had going on.

My partner who had joined with me at the very beginning of my journey was no longer a part of our company. She wanted to spend time with her grandchildren, and, although her heart was still in it, her mind was not. The battle raging in her own mind would prove to be one she could not fight while still working. For her, her family, and our company's best interest, we decided to part ways so her full focus could be on healing.

Because my team had already lived through the withdrawal of one owner, they seemingly had some unresolved abandonment issues that my lack of presence stirred up.

By God's grace, after the parting of my original partner, but before the expansion, I had accumulated two new partners, Jo and Emily. Jo was a high-level stylist within our Eastside company and would, therefore, be the one in charge at that location. Emily was a former work colleague of mine from "the other salon" and she would be the one in charge of Westside.

* * *

Once again God would redeem a troubled past. I had built my position up in the other salon from front desk night support to salon manager. I hired, fired, set schedules, and did payroll when the owner was away. I could do, and often did do, all the things!

I had hired Emily as a front desk team member, though she was young and often came to work with her eye make-up from the night before smudged under her eyes and still smelling a bit of alcohol.

She was good at her job and great with our guests. After nearly two years (and after I had left to be a stay-at-home mom), Emily would leave in a staged coup, with a few other employees, to go to another salon (the grass is always greener, right?)

She would spend the next few years becoming an alcoholic, becoming sober, becoming a wife, and becoming a mom before our paths would cross again.

When she first reached out to me for an interview at Sorella Westside, I was skeptical. Her honesty and transparency about what she had gone through since we had last worked together reminded me of why I got into owning a business in the first place: to be able to show others the love that Christ had shown me. We became fast friends and then business partners.

The trouble with the team and their connection with Emily, as the authority figure, was that she was new. In their eyes, she had yet to put in the time and earn the right. Every decision Emily made was met with criticism. No matter how good she was, to them, she was not good enough.

I remember having a conversation with one of my longest employed team members. She was honest with me about how she didn't trust the people (Emily and Jo) I had chosen to partner with. She felt as though they were taking advantage of me and were pulling the wool over my eyes.

I responded to her as I would several more times over our eight years together, "Do you trust *me*?" She didn't have to trust them yet, she just had to trust me. With tear-filled eyes, she nodded yes.

With Jo as an authority figure, the trouble was that she had been just like them. She was a stylist, a buddy. Just because she bought into the company didn't mean that relationship should change in their view, but it did change. The closer Jo and I worked together on developing her leadership skills, the further she grew apart from her buddies. Any improvement in her life or advancement in her career was met with eye-rolls and whispers.

Although it never surprises me, I am always saddened when friends drift apart because one decides to invest in her personal growth, make choices to expand her career instead of partying, chooses to have conversations over ideas instead of over people, or chooses to have a positive attitude over a negative one. Once this shift begins, two outcomes can happen:

1. The other friend is inspired by her willingness to grow and wants to support and encourage her in any way she can. She's proud of her for overcoming the difficulties of her past, making the hard choices, knowing that one day she can and will create her own path of growth and enlightenment.

2. Her friend feels threatened by her growth and this new, contradictory way of thinking. Accusations such as, "You don't know what you're talking about" become common. If she sees her friend stumble over a growth hurdle, she views her as a fraud. She is the first to criticize any achievement made and is always looking for ways to watch her fail. Envying her subconsciously and disliking her consciously are far easier than putting in the effort and hard work to grow out of a current level of thinking. No matter how miserable she is (although she will not admit it) in her current conditions and circumstances, her fear of change—of the unknown—still holds more power over her. Until she is sick and tired of being sick and tired, being the victim of all that happens to and around her, and being the only reason she is not achieving more out life, she will pity those trying to improve and remain bound.

You see, the thing about praying for God to bring the people into your business that he wants there ... he does just that. I have yet to have a team member that had his or her life together, nor have I had one that hasn't had a troubled past, or even present!

In the past eight years, I have employed men and women who have come to me claiming to have experienced the following:

- Trauma
- Abuse (physical, mental, emotional)
- Neglect
- Addiction (drugs and/or alcohol)
- Abandonment
- Prostitution
- Adultery

- Divorce
- Attempted Suicide
- Mental Illness
- Custody Battles
- Lies/Betrayal

I have yet to have a team member with an *easy* life. Not once has there been an employee that didn't need growth, guidance, and support. Not one that didn't need to see a glimpse of what Christ's unconditional and redeeming love looks like—lived out.

Don't get me wrong, I am by no means an angelic, no problems, stumble-free, have it all figured out kinda gal. I am an imperfect person redeemed by a perfect God. And although I am not perfect at it, I live to love people as Christ does.

I just have a whole lot more "Julie" that gets in the way when people make unwise choices!

Emily has to constantly remind me to "put my sword away." And by "sword," she is referring to my burning, instinctive drive for justice. Emily is the caramel to my salt. Apart, we tend to be too intense for certain tastes, but together we balance each other out.

My saltiness may not be quite what Jesus was referring to in his Sermon on the Mount when he refers to his disciples as "the salt of the earth," in Matthew 5:13 (NIV), but I'm working on it.

I love Al Capone's quote that says, "Do not mistake my kindness for weakness, I am kind to everyone, but when someone is unkind to me, weak is not what you are going to remember about me."[3] That's me in a nutshell, I guess. I love Jesus and I cuss a little ... I quote scripture and gangsters!

After a year of trying to make it work with two separate locations, our lease at the eastside location was coming to end, so we decided to go ahead and merge the two. I was able to get out of my lease early by paying off the remaining five months' rent at a reduced rate.

However, since we were still dealing with other debt, I had to put the remainder of what was owed on our personal credit card (insert face palm emoji).

Another challenge I faced, having opened a salon based on my naïve understanding of contracts and loans, I was in my SBA loan for ten years.

We would be closing the eastside location in year five, leaving five years' worth of payments remaining.

We looked into filing bankruptcy, but apparently, when you sign as the personal guarantor of a loan, you are held responsible for paying the debt load if the company is unable to.

We then thought I could file personal bankruptcy, but because I was on the mortgage of our home, it would make our home fair game to satisfy the loan. So even though I never signed my house for collateral, it could still be used as such.

To complicate matters further, our home was now being used as collateral for our westside location. Oh, crap!

* * *

The thing about being in a crappy situation is that as much as you cry about it, as much as you worry about it, as much as you whine and complain about it not being fair, the truth is you are in the crap, and the more you focus on the crap and all that surrounds it, the stinkier it gets and the less likely you are to see the solution.

I also refer to being in crap as "the trenches."

When you are in over your head in the sloppy, deep mud of the trenches; it's raining, and you have just lost a shoe, and it feels like everything and/or everyone is against you; remember that "the power that resides in you is greater than the power of the circumstances that threaten your joy!" —Carly Fiorina.[4]

SIDE NOTE: *There is an air of skepticism that surrounds believers claiming "personal power."*

For example, some people think that talking about the "power within" means putting their own strength over God's—that they don't actually need Jesus because they have "personal power." Some say that if a proclaimed believer refers to the "power within" or "personal power," then she must not truly be a believer. I feel the air around this subject is cloudy and pungent. It's because I am a believer that I can confidently claim the power within me ... because I know where that power comes from! The moment I became a believer, the holy power of a living God, through the Holy Spirit, dwelled within me and nothing is more personal than that.

Obstacles are opportunities to grow, not excuses to quit! It is in the tough times that our character is revealed.

The importance of personal growth is to daily, intentionally build your character during the day to day when your emotions are in a more stable place.

If you wait until sh*t hits the fan to build your character, your emotions are high. And when emotions are high, intelligence is low. That's not just a great saying, it is scientific fact.[5]

Life is hard and full of trench-y, uncomfortable, crappy and sometimes downright sh*tty situations, but as Susan David says: "Discomfort is the price of admission to a meaningful *life!"*[6] *I have yet to be inspired to live into my best life by someone who has never gone through any of the hard times. The stories of encouragement that oxygenate my soul are those that have endured, triumphed, and had victory over the hard.*

Although our financial struggles would carry on for many more years, our team culture was improving, and we were experiencing higher sales months than ever before. Getting to see team members buy new cars, move out of a parent's house, buy a new home, afford insurance, travel, advance their education ... seeing them able to live into their potential brought me so much joy that I was willing to forgo my paychecks when we had tighter months.

My friendship with Emily and Jo would grow deeper and become invaluable to me. In fact, we would get matching tattoos of three connected hearts with 16:3 along the side—Proverbs 16:3 (CEV), the verse on which I had established the salon years ago, reads, "Commit your plans to the Lord so that they will succeed." We did the same for our friendship! A friendship that would endure the hurricane to come.

CHAPTER NINE

The Disturbance

I have heard your prayers and seen your tears;
I will heal you.

—2 Kings 20:5 NIV

I'm sure you have heard about, and maybe even experienced, "the perfect storm" in your own life. If you're not sure what I mean, the perfect storm is a particularly bad or critical state of affairs, arising from a number of negative and unpredictable factors.

I always visualize the perfect storm as a hurricane. Hurricanes are the most violent storms on earth, they are like engines that require warm air as fuel.

Meteorologists have divided the development of a hurricane into four stages: tropical disturbance, tropical depression, tropical storm, and a full-fledged hurricane. My perfect storm would likewise have four levels of development.

The Disturbance was brought about within my own body. When Jack was one, I decided to get breast implants. I had always had a larger chest, but breastfeeding my kiddos sucked all the "meat" out of them.

My once-full bosom now resembled deflated balloons. I wanted to get implants to put back what had been lost. I wanted my clothes to fit right again, I wanted to not have a moment of sadness every time I glanced at my naked body in the mirror, as I got in the shower.

Did I still love my body and appreciate all it was able to accomplish carrying and nursing my two children? Absolutely! Was I still saddened by my deflated breasts? Absolutely.

But eight years after implants, I developed a severe capsulation of my right breast and suffered from breast implant illness (BII).

At this point, I had a grade-four contracture. My breast was visibly distorted and extremely painful to the touch. I had a general chronic pain that felt like a ten-pound softball had been shoved in my breast. I had two firm bubbles, about a thumbs length apart, at the top of my breast where the contracture had squeezed the implant so tightly that I was no longer able to wear a regular bra without severe discomfort. I had to find sports bras that were supportive, soft, and had enough material in the front to mask the bubbles that made it look like I had three nipples!

My main symptoms of BII were chest and breast pain, chronic pain, unexplained fatigue, heat at the site, the general feeling of malaise, and hormonal changes. My hormonal changes, however, could have also stemmed from my hysterectomy and removal of one ovary.

In my situation, it was hard to tell what came first, the chicken (implants) or the egg (hysterectomy)? Were my implants a contributing factor in my hormonal changes adding to the list of reasons for needing a hysterectomy?

After carrying quadruplets, my insides were all kinds of messed up. My doctor said my uterus looked like a baked potato that had been smashed with a hammer. I not only had endometriosis (which I had always had), but I now had uterine enhanced Myometrial Adenomyosis and Vascularity.

Basically, the lining of my uterus broke through the muscle wall, and because of how far my uterus stretched during pregnancy, I had acquired increased vascularity and arteriovenous malformations, all causing prolonged, more frequent, painful, and flooding type periods.

In other words, my uterus was destroyed. Hence, the hysterectomy!

Because I was preoccupied with my life and my business, I swept all my symptoms under the rug, only to learn that if you do not take time for your health, you will be forced to take time for your sickness.

As I was experiencing my own storm, my brother Brian was experiencing his own personal perfect storm. I just happened to be caught up in it because he was living with me at the time.

* * *

I had always wanted to be my brother's friend.

I am the youngest by three years. He and my sister are just 22 months apart and always had a closer bond growing up.

My sister was five years older than me and didn't want to have anything to do with her annoying, younger sister. Thankfully, all this would change when she went to college.

My brother would play with me because I was athletic and my sister was not; however, it never really felt like he liked me ... more like he tolerated me to have someone to play basketball with.

Brian, like my dad, is an attractive, charismatic guy, whom everyone enjoys being around. He was never short on friends or the ability to make friends. Like the stereotypical middle child, Brian possessed traits of being the peacemaker.

Sociable, loyal, and empathetic, he would also prove to have the 50% of hereditary contributing factors in known alcoholics. This disease would cost him his marriage, full custody of his girls, and almost his life. I will not go into full details of Brian's journey, as it is his story to tell, and it would be a bestseller if ever he decided to put it on paper. I will simply share the part of his story that took place while he was living with me.

Having six kids, I tend to always be looking down, not meta-phorically, but actually physically looking down because my kids are all below chest level. Any time we're together in public, my attention is drawn downward. I have had people think of me as mean and self-absorbed because I failed to recognize them when I was out with my kids.

Truth be told, after the whole circumcision debacle, when I was out with my kids, I was full-on mama-bear! Their safety mattered to me more than the opinions of others.

My kids are not an excuse for my lack of attention toward my brother, or anyone else for that matter.

I would like to think that I just did not see him getting sick, that I did not notice how yellow he was, or that he had gained 43 pounds, but it very well could be that I didn't want to see it.

I was juggling enough, and to add another ball in the air would have sent everything else crashing down. I focused on the balls I had in play until I couldn't ignore what I was seeing anymore.

Brian, like me, has always been hot natured. Even in the cold-

est of winter, we both sleep with our ceiling fans on, plus an additional fan pointed straight at our face, so when I started seeing him head to toe in sweats, pulling blankets on himself with his teeth chattering, I knew something was wrong.

Three months prior, we had all recognized Brian had still been drinking, and his body was failing him because of it. Three years prior to that, after going through an outpatient rehab process, Brian had become sober. But like most, when life became too stressful, his bad habits and harmful ways of thinking, left him grasping for an "easy" form of comfort.

He reasoned that because, this time, he would not be drinking liquor, he would be okay ... he could handle it. His choice of easy comfort would have consequences that would prove to be harder than anything he had ever endured before.

Here he was in October, having gotten sober in the past, determined to do it on his own this time. He wanted to not only be sober, he wanted to be healthy again. He looked up diets for healthy liver function. I had given him a box of my detox tea and cleanse supplements that I had ordered to do a 30-day healthy living cleanse.

These products were all-natural and to a relatively healthy individual would offer the needed results; however, Brian's organs were failing and, therefore, these normally gentle cleansing ingredients would prove to act on his organs in the way that sandpaper would rip into a silk blouse!

He developed an infection in his lymph nodes and had extreme swelling under his chin. I immediately took him to the doctor. Even knowing all his symptoms, his doctor prescribed him Biaxin, a medication to treat the infection. This particular medication, in combination with everything else happening within his body, precipitated a harsh reaction, resulting in Stevens-Johnsons Syndrome.

I had left for work on Wednesday morning with Brian bundled up in the living room recliner. All day, I wrestled with what to do. He kept saying he was fine, just fighting a cough (which he did have). I knew in my gut he was not okay.

At work, I told Emily about how he had been acting the past several days, and she immediately called her sister-in-law, an ER nurse, who recommended he be seen. Brian had a check-up scheduled on Friday with the doctor that had prescribed him the Biaxin, so she said we could wait until then, but if I felt he needed to be seen sooner, to go ahead and bring him in.

I called Brian as I was leaving work, and he said he would rather just wait until Friday, as he didn't have insurance and couldn't afford a hospital visit. Driving home I prayed:

> "Lord, I need you! I don't even know what words to pray right now. I am afraid for my brother's life. Lord, I don't know what is happening within his body, but you do! He is my big brother! He has always been the strong one, but Lord, he is broken right now. Please guide me to make the right decision about his care. Remove my own weakness and insecurity and help me see him and his needs clearly. And Lord, please let me catch every green light so I can get to him faster! Amen."

I still had that little girl inside of me that just wanted her big brother to like her, and she was trying to reason with me. Thankfully, God silenced that voice, and when I got home I took him to the ER. That day he would be admitted into the ICU where he would remain for 13 days, fighting for his life.

I visited him every day; some days I could only stay for an hour, but I didn't want him to be alone. I wanted him to know how loved he was, how important he was, how he was a precious child of God who was still alive for a purpose!

I wanted him to know how much his little girls needed their daddy. My mom was great to bring pictures they had colored *to hang in his room so he could feel their presence. Since he was in the ICU, he and his ex-wife had agreed it best that his girls did not see him like that.*

Once out of the hospital, Brian was ready to live his life with an attitude of gratitude. He started easing back into exercising and joined a Bible study. It was in that Bible study one evening that his new hematology doctor would call him and tell him his recent hemoglobin count was dangerously low. He needed to head back to the ER, and in no way could he drive himself.

Unlike my low hemoglobin scare, his was not caused by a blood draw from an arm with an IV in it. Brian was bleeding internally, and this hospital stay would last six days and require multiple blood transfusions.

Brian had survived the new year in seemingly good health and was back to living a healthy lifestyle. Back in December, when he first went into the hospital, we noticed little spots on his chest that looked like small broken capillaries. That was the least of his issues—issues not addressed until a month later when those small red bumps would turn into huge red patches of blisters and sores all over his body.

This would be when he was diagnosed with Stevens-Johnson Syndrome or SJS (a toxic epidermal necrolysis that is a very severe reaction, most commonly triggered by medications, that causes skin tissue to die—necrosis—and detach).[7]

This syndrome would leave him unable to walk for several days, as the blisters on his feet were debilitatingly painful. Every night I would ease his feet into a foot-soak of warm water and Epsom salts. I would then lift each swollen foot, careful not to rupture the larger blisters, while placing them on my lap. I would then, carefully, with a sterilized needle, drain the blisters and wrap them.

Now, almost two years later, he still has light scarring all over his body and has not regained full feeling in his feet. Although the scars remain, they do not speak as loud as the lessons learned.

Brian conveys his message to be one of humility, hope, and gratitude. He says: "When it's time to speak up ... do it, no matter how hard it is, and don't wait. Your life may very well depend on it. Don't fear the shame or the judgment of others ... it's false ... scary, but false! No matter how hard the situation, family and true friends will be there to help. If you are alive today, it is for a purpose, and embracing an attitude of gratitude will give you drive to keep moving forward! And remember, at the end of the day ... God is for you!" Brian's perfect storm of medical conditions was a humbling reminder of perspective.

✳ ✳ ✳

Remembering my brother's story, I knew I had to pay attention to what was happening in my body. I knew I wasn't right; I knew I needed help. Once again my health would get placed on the back burner as my "tropical disturbance" was about to gain speed, turning into a "tropical depression."

CHAPTER TEN

The Depression

*And the rain fell, and the floods came, and the winds blew
and beat on that house, but it did not fall, because it had
been founded on the rock.*

—Matthew 7:25 TLV

I had a hard time praying for miracles anymore after my
dad died.

Every time since then, when conditions and circumstances
called me to my knees in prayer, I had met them with doubt
... lack of faith that God would work another miracle in my
life.

I prayed so hard for my dad's miracle ... I pleaded with God
to let my father be the first one to survive Alzheimer's. He
was only 63 years old, still strong and vibrant. If anyone
could physically handle a comeback ... *Lord, let it be my dad.*

He died four days later.

Maybe we only get so many miracles in a lifetime. Maybe I
had already used mine all up?

He had blessed me with my six kids, a husband who honors

the Lord and our vows, a company that was built on God's grace, determination, and souls who needed second chances.

I also had to consider that in a week's time I had prayed both for the miracle of my father's healing and the mercy to let him die. With wavering emotions, I suppose it is best that God is working for the good of those who love him, despite my input.

We had known my dad was experiencing dementia-like symptoms, but the tests had yet to confirm Alzheimer's.

In 2013 his condition was classified as mild cognitive impairment with diffuse brain atrophy. He would constantly ask what the time was, he was easily confused, and he would get turned around while driving. He also developed a tremor in his hands.

Before the diagnosis, we naively thought, perhaps, he had been drinking or abusing prescription drugs, as having four back surgeries in the past, addiction to opioids wasn't a far-fetched thought. We even went as far as checking him into an outpatient recovery program.

I sat in the counselor's office at the Recovery Center, tears falling, pleading with my dad to get help. He put his hand on top of mine, which was resting on my trembling leg. Hoping to calm his youngest daughter, he looked at me with tears in his eyes and said, "Okay."

He explained to the counselor that he was not suffering from addiction of any kind, but since neither he nor anyone else could explain his hand tremor and foggy memory, he agreed to get help.

As horrible as addiction would have been, I would gladly have taken that over what was to come, and I don't make that claim lightly, as I know the devastating effects addiction can have on a person and their loved ones.

I hate that I did not believe my dad.

Alcoholism has always been so prevalent in our family that it just made sense. I hate that his time in the recovery center was a waste! I hate that I could have been using that time to make precious memories with my dad, instead of sitting in the Wednesday night Family Support meeting.

My dad aspired to do everything he could to love, protect, and support his family. When money was tight (as it was most of my growing up years), he took on multiple jobs to make ends meet.

He swept peanuts off the floor, after hours, of a roadhouse-type restaurant.

He delivered newspapers in the early hours of the morning, and a few other odds and ends jobs.

One night I had asked my dad if he would wake me up when he left for his paper route, so I could ride along with him. I had to bundle up extra warm as we would ride with the car windows down.

The simple joy of spending time with my dad tossing newspapers from a moving car sounds ridiculous, but that memory will be with me forever: the crisp air, the smell of the morning dew on the grass, the black smudges the newspaper left on my hands, and the sound of the Bee Gees playing. Looking back, I treasure that memory, but at the time, I never talked about riding with my dad.

I went to an elite college prep school that I was able to attend on scholarship assistance from my mom's teaching benefits. I never felt my life was *good enough.* I felt ashamed of not having enough money, the fancy cars, the new clothes, the exotic trips, the 10,000+ square-foot homes, the mom who stayed at home making perfect meals, and the dad who was a brilliant surgeon and easily paid for all the activities my siblings and I wanted to do.

I was young, stupid, and caught up in the devil's playground of comparison. In hindsight, I can see how truly blessed we were. My parents were still married and in love, and they loved us fully.

I had meaningful friendships (one still holding strong over 25 years later and eight states apart), my mom had summers off to stay home with us. We never had to deal with any form of abuse within our family.

I excelled in sports, swimming, volleyball, track, basketball— really any sport with the exception of soccer, where my coach told me I was great at kicking the ball ... as long as it wasn't moving! I did well in school, despite never truly applying myself. We didn't have everything we wanted, but we had everything we needed.

There are times I wish I could have those moments back, the moments that I wasted caring about what the other kids thought of me—the moments I wasted not feeling pretty enough, smart enough, rich enough, good enough—to have back all the hours I wasted concerning myself with all the things out of my control.

Today, if I got all that time back, I would have the time needed to fold and put away all my family's laundry, and that is saying something!

✳ ✳ ✳

I have to be careful wishing for change in my past, as it took all those moments, all that pain, to help shape my perspective into what it is now.

They were like ugly, misshapen seeds ... despite what they started out looking like, once planted in soil, given water, and light ... they yielded the same beautiful flower as the seeds that appeared to have everything going for them from the beginning.

So much of the happiness you find in life is directly related to the effort of the perspective you choose to have. I love the quote from Joyce Meyer that says, "You may have been given a cactus, but you don't have to sit on it!"[8]

I also love the theme from the movie Trolls *which colorfully, and with a great soundtrack explains, "Happiness isn't something you put inside you. It's already there!"—Princess Poppy.[9]*

＊ ＊ ＊

Although looking back is a slippery slope for me, I know that experience will only take me so far. It is an evaluated experience that makes all the difference if I am to grow into my potential and be the woman my daddy always encouraged me to be, the woman God created, with purpose and passion. I have to spend time in reflection and evaluation. Doing so is easier now that we are a year out from his death. I am able to see a clearer and broader picture.

After my dad got out of rehab, nothing changed for the better. Over the next few years, we would witness more confusion and irritability. He was becoming more irritable with himself, forgetting things, always hearing people say, "I just told you that, don't you remember?" And we were becoming more irritable with him for asking the same question repeatedly and getting confused during a conversation.

One would think it was easy to ignore or not let it become bothersome, and although maybe it "should" have been, it wasn't. I had a hard time being around my dad during what would have been the last year of his life.

By early 2017, we had a PET scan done confirming a definitive diagnosis of Early Onset Alzheimer's. Dad would only live 18 months beyond that diagnosis. I no longer recognized the man in front of me as my dad.

Alzheimer's doesn't just cause one to forget his place in a conversation, what time it is, where he is driving to; no, Alzheimer's causes one to forget how to come up with words needed in a conversation, forget how to draw the face of a clock and the numbers needed to go on it, forget the mechanics of how to drive, forget how to eat soup, forget how to wash properly.

He could no longer reason or plan. He was unable to show restraint or empathy along with other heart-wrenching truths. There were so many times towards the end where I saw my father as a lost child, and instead of being a better caregiver, I would get irritated that I had *another* child to care for. It wasn't just *me* feeling that way. My whole family was exhausted.

There were many middle-of-the-night manhunts trying to find where my dad had wandered. One early morning around 3:00 a.m., both my sister and brother took separate cars to drive a five-mile perimeter around my parents' apartment complex while my mom searched the grounds around their unit.

Dad often liked to try to find cars that were unlocked to climb into and go! Karen found my dad in the woods just outside their apartment complex. She pulled off the road yelling for him to come to her. After falling down the steep hill of wet leaves in the dark, Karen got to her feet and reached my dad.

The joy of finding him was quickly replaced by anger and frustration after her fall. Dad was so confused as to why she was upset. He thought she had just come to visit him and "the people." The people referred to the hallucination he had of the dozens of friends, former employees, or strangers who lived in the woods. After Karen put him in the car, he asked her if she had brought him food.

While I did have a few heartfelt moments of kindness and compassion, they were few and far between. In these moments, I would get a glimpse of my dad, not the Alzheimer's patient.

Looking into my dad's sea-blue eyes during those glimpses, I could see him! My dad, the man God had created, the man that loved my mother unconditionally.

I could see the heaviness he felt, living with a mind he no longer had control over. I could see his eagerness to return to his family. I could see his unfailing love and awe he had for his sweetheart. I could see his grit to fight the disease. I could see his sadness for the loss of his future with his family and watching all eleven grandkids grow up. I could see his frustration with not recognizing an old friend. I could see his sorrow in not fulfilling the life he desired to live with my mom.

His smile covered a multitude of emotions, but his eyes told all. My dad was being held captive by his mind, and it was killing him.

※ ※ ※

The Deep Sadness

My 34th birthday started out as a normal day.

I went to work, ate some delicious Mexican with my partners, and enjoyed my day. Later that afternoon, my stomach began to turn. I thought, surely it was the Mexican and it would settle. Not long after that thought, I began to sweat and my mouth began to water—never a good sign.

I was determined to "mind over matter" this stomach thing; I did not have time to get sick. And it was my birthday! After running to the bathroom, where the matter completely dominated my mind, I cried on the cold tile floor with my head resting on a porcelain pillow.

Just as I gathered my strength to stand, I heard Ashton (now age three) briefly scream, vomit, and scream again. OH NO! The throw-up bug had officially infested our home! Happy friggin birthday to me!

The next day, Friday, Matt stayed home from work, as I was too weak to mommy. This bug was no 24-hour or one-and-done type bug, it was a mutated beast that had no mercy.

I was able to function by Saturday—in spite of my dehydration headache and shaky limbs—because I had no choice.

My sister had called and said she was on her way, with dad, to the hospital. The facility he was in had called and said he was wandering into other patients' rooms in his underwear and socks.

He was speaking nonsense and causing unspeakable chaos. The facility told my sister that they could not handle our father and that she needed to come get him.

This was not the first facility that could not handle my dad. Just five days prior, I had walked in to visit my dad at the original senior living facility. He had resided there for only three days, having escaped several times. Just that morning, he was found by the mailman, a mile down the road.

The nurses just laughed and made light of how much energy my dad had and how no one can keep tabs on him. After much research, this facility was the one my mom decided on as it was state-of-the-art, had cognitive care, and offered advanced care for Alzheimer's and dementia patients.

Another plus, it was not a lock-down facility, which allowed him the freedom to walk to the various places on the property and not be confined to an 8x10 room within a hallway that just makes a giant circle and has no end. Unfortunately, this type of facility was great for Alzheimer's patients who are in a wheelchair or don't walk much; this type of facility was NOT for my dad.

Two nights prior, the director had awakened my mom in the middle of the night with a phone call saying my dad had escaped and she, her staff, and the police were searching in the cold dark night, down by the lake, trying to find him. No need to be asleep to have a nightmare. One of the main reasons we agreed to put my dad in a facility was that he was wandering too much in the middle of the night and my mom just couldn't keep up. This facility had assured us that they could properly care for him.

After the nurse laughed off the mailman incident, I got two inches away from her face and said, "My father's life was in danger! He was walking down a very busy highway, and not one of you even knew he was gone. I need to speak to the director right now."

The nurse apologized and said that the director wasn't there. I then told her, "Well, you better call her, and she can talk to me on the phone or come meet me here. I'll wait."

Moments later, I had the director on the phone. I told her that if she could not guarantee my father's safety that I would be leaving her facility and taking my father with me. She agreed that their care was inadequate for my father's needs. So to my house we went.

I called my mom on the way home and told her what I had done. She was frustrated, not so much with me and my boldness, but more with the situation. She now had to find somewhere for him to go where he could not escape, and that meant a lock-down facility, with the small rooms and the never-ending hallway. I told her I would handle finding him a place. She and my brother just needed to go to the old facility to get his things.

Home with me was busy but do-able. My dad actually slept a lot that afternoon, which allowed me the time to make several phone calls about his care. When the kids got home from school, we all went on a walk together.

I watched him stroll down the street holding Bradlee's little hand. As she looked up at her "Dude" (my dad's choice of names instead of "Grandpa") while singing, something inside told me to take a photo. The light streaming in through the trees, the sweet sound of my kid's made up lyrics, and the smile on my dad's face. It's like I knew this kind of precious moment would never happen again.

Having gone for a walk, my dad functioned more normally because he was physically tired. His brain would be active, but his body wasn't as willing to participate, which made caring for him a bit easier. That evening, as he fumbled through eating his dinner telling me nonsense stories, I had to look up and smile. Not because I was happy to be with my dad, but because it was the only thing keeping the tears from falling.

After I gave him a bath (I had to use a bath bomb to color the water, so he wouldn't be afraid, as oftentimes Alzheimer's patients fear water because they can't see or understand it), I had to have Matt help him get out of the tub and dry off.

I have asked much of my husband over the years, but this time, this favor, evoked all kinds of emotions within me. Matt had already lost his father and was now helping me care for mine. It didn't seem fair. He was more than willing to do it and all with a smile on his face. He loved me and my dad and wanted to help care for him. As Matt dressed my dad for bed, I booby-trapped the door because we needed to be able to hear my dad when he awoke ready to wander.

I used two of my running medallions to fasten around the door so that when it opened, they would clang together. I also placed a metal bat at the front door so it would create a loud bang against the hardwood floors if the door were to open.

I was ready. I was not ready, however, for what would actually happen that night. I had just relaxed enough to finally fall asleep when I heard the clanging of the metals and ran to my dad's room at 2:00 a.m. He was standing in the doorway shaking and crying. I was unprepared to see him like that. He had been having a hallucination that "the people" were attacking me and he couldn't get out of his bed because he was scared, but he had to help me! He got out of his bed to fight "the people," but I was gone. He just kept shaking and crying saying, "They were hurting you and I couldn't help you! I couldn't get to you." My heart sank.

No smile could stop my tears, as I said, "I'm okay, Dad! I'm safe, you are safe, we are okay. Look, Dad, I'm right here. I'm safe! You did a good job, I'm okay!"

I just held him for a moment until he caught his breath. I asked him if he wanted to lie back down or if he would rather go into the living room with me and watch a show. Still visibly shaken, he chose the show. Once the show started, his brain switched and he was talking to me like nothing happened, just laughing at the TV and asking for some peanut M&M's.

I stayed awake with my dad, thinking of all the ways I could make his living with us work … I would find a way, so he didn't have to go to a lock-down facility. It was a long night.

The next day was an unusually busy kind, several pick-ups, drop-offs, I had to go to the store, just a lot of going. The problem with the go, go, go, is that Dad's mind would enter a manic-type state.

*On the way to taking Jack to swim practice, the kids asked to listen to the theme song from **Space Jam**. It is a very upbeat, catchy song and they love to bounce to it. Within the first few seconds of the song playing, my dad became increasingly agitated.*

He started to pull and grab at his shirt and seatbelt. He was gritting his teeth, closing his eyes, and exhaling deeply through his nostrils. I was instantly alarmed and turned the music to the Beatles' "Here Comes The Sun." The melody calmed my dad and he settled. I, however, did not.

The ride back home consisted of easy tunes and me calmly demanding my kids keep quiet. Campbell knew something was wrong and tried to keep the four three-year-olds calm. Once home, we got my dad situated in the living room watching one of his favorite shows while I started dinner.

My mom had met us at the house to join us for dinner. My dad would always light up whenever he saw his sweetheart.

My mom had gone to sit with Bradlee in our other living room when I heard Walker crying. A toy had been taken from him and he was whining about it on the landing above the two stairs that led down to the living room where my dad was watching TV.

I was still in the kitchen and told Walker to hush and go play, but before I could say more, out of the corner of my eye I could see my dad swoop Walker up in his arms and storm off. I followed my dad in confusion.

"Dad, what are you doing?" I questioned.

He turned his head over his shoulder, his face contorted in anger, "I have to make the noise stop!" he said while squeezing Walker.

The noise had stopped; Walker was terrified and couldn't move.

"Dad, look at me ... put Walker down. You are okay! DAD ... put ... Walker ... down!" I demanded.

Not breaking eye contact, I saw whatever "demon" that was possessing my father release.

His face softened and he gently set Walker down and walked back into the living room. I had never seen anything like that before. This was what my mom saw every night when he would become increasingly agitated and show aggression towards her.

I knew at that moment, he could not stay with us. His mind was broken. Putting my kids' lives and even my dad's best interest on the line—just to prove that I could care for him, that I would find a way to make it work—was selfish.

He needed care that none of us were equipped to offer.

The next morning I would drive my dad, while my mom and sister followed, to the lock-down facility over an hour away. Leaving my dad that day was one of the hardest things I had ever done.

Sitting outside in my car, with tear-filled eyes, I watched my dad walking the endless hallway, looking scared as he searched for his sweetheart, no doubt. The facts were: he needed to be there, and he needed constant supervision. But the facts weren't the whole truth.

The truth was, my dad needed his family. Deep down I knew the moment we left, he gave up. If he couldn't be with his family, he didn't want to be at all. Five days later, my sister was obliged to take him back to the hospital, where he would never leave.

When he first arrived at the hospital, he was rambling non-sense. His eyes would, for the most part, remain shut. As much odd behavior as we had seen from my dad, this was a whole new level.

Even the doctors thought for sure he had something else going on. Some kind of infection? Had he had a stroke? They ran ALL the tests. My dad became so agitated, he had to be both chemically and physically restrained ... yet he fought! He would sit up in his bed, eyes and fists clenched and try to physically fight while yelling obscenities.

My dad was never big on cursing, and he was always funny, congenial, and cooperative whenever he had been in hospitals (which was frequent with his four previous back surgeries). In fact, nurses always complimented him as being their favorite patient. But not this guy. I didn't know who I was watching come unglued, but it was not my father. I just kept thinking— this must be what demonic possession is like.

Finally, after a third cocktail of tranquilizers, my dad was out.

Early Sunday, my dad would be diagnosed as having terminal aggression. He was dying, yet his mind was still firing. He would go into hospice care Sunday and never come out.

He stayed on a heavy and steady dose of morphine and valium. Just before the time for his next dose, he would moan and lift his arms a few inches off the bed in an effort to still fight (although he had given up his fight to control his mind the day we dropped him off, his mind was at war).

The days crept by slowly, I was still weak from having been sick, and I was emotionally exhausted.

Each day I would go to the hospital, praying for a miracle or God's mercy to take him home. Neither came.

Tuesday, I sat at his side and wiped the foam that continuously oozed from his nose. I held his increasingly cold and clammy hands. He maintained a high fever throughout the day. The staff assured us that all these symptoms were a part of the dying process, and that, although we were hurting for him, he was not in any pain.

I spent the afternoon alone with him, engulfed with a deep sadness, where I prayed, talked to him, played his favorite songs, and wrote the lyrics to Chris Tomlin's song "Home" and put them over his headboard. They begin: "This world is not what it was meant to be ... All this pain, all this suffering ... There's a better place waiting for me ... In Heaven."[10]

*My dad would finally go **home** two days later, after only five days in hospice care, exactly one week after my birthday. We will forever celebrate my dad's "Heaven Gotcha" day!*

✳ ✳ ✳

Having worked through depression after my miscarriage, I was no stranger to the symptoms when they started forming after my dad died. I had waded out into the metaphorical deep, dark water and it was beginning to rise. I was caught up in being busy with life (husband, kids, the business), being frustrated with how my dad died, being angry that he was only 63 years old, and being overwhelmed at having to pick up his remains from the crematorium.

✳ ✳ ✳

I called the funeral home director to ask when my father's remains would be available. He assured me it would be later that same afternoon. I was already discouraged that the beautiful University of Georgia (UGA) urn I had ordered for his remains had not shown up yet, which meant I could not bring it with me to have the funeral home put his remains in it, and, therefore, I would have to do it myself. CRINGE!

I arrived at the funeral home around 4:00 p.m., knowing that would have allowed for plenty of time. I had two of my kids with me and wanted the process to run as smoothly as possible. I checked in with the front desk and was taken aback by her response, "Oh! Oh, Ms. Kirkland ... ummmmm, well ... hold on for me just a moment."

A mortician came around the corner 20 minutes later, and, with no regard to bedside manner, said, "Yes, Ms. Kirkland, the cremains are still hot! I mean, I can get them for you if you want, but they are not cooled down yet."

CRINGE CRINGE CRINGE!!!

I said no thank you and that I would return tomorrow. I grabbed my kids and literally ran out of there. Having to pick up a beloved from a funeral home while having your daddy referred to as "Hot Cremains." How horrible!

✳ ✳ ✳

I just kept shoving those depression warning symptoms deeper and deeper down. I have since learned that suppression leads to depression.

No one else can deal with your emotions; although, others may get caught in the wake of them. The thoughts and energy driving your emotions is 100% on you to deal with.

As blunt and often harsh as this truth is, no matter how you got into your conditions and circumstances ... even if everything happens to you and you played no part in where you are now, the only one that can get you out is YOU!

Don't hear what I'm not saying—I am not saying that you won't need support, or counsel, or medication to aid you in the process—what I am saying is that the dark cloud of depression can be pierced with the love and light of Jesus.

If you have not heard anything in this book up until now, hear this: God is for you! He wants to fight for you! He wants you to claim victory in his name! He came to give you an abundant life filled with joy, peace, and hope. And although it is given freely, the abundant life was purchased at the highest price.

The only requirement to receive it is believing and confessing it to be true. Sounds simple, right?

We tend to over-complicate the simplest things. That is why God calls us to have childlike faith. Adults are excellent at compiling complicated excuses as to why we can't do something or why it won't work. Our fact-driven nature often overrides our faith-filled purpose.

Think about this as if you were trying to sell a house—when the realtor comes to take pictures, you are told to put the clutter away.

More clutter causes confusion and distraction. Even when you think you have gotten all the obvious distractions out of the way, there could still be pieces that you have become desensitized to.

When we tried to sell our house, we decluttered like mad! It would take me a solid, uninterrupted, kids-out-of-the-house three hours to put away all the stuff that might distract a potential buyer; yet, oftentimes they would get distracted by the little boys' room where the three matching beds sat in a row, or the picture on the wall of quadruplet babies, or the fact that we had to turn our laundry room into an extended pantry and our garage into a larger living room with a bigger laundry room built within it, or within the laundry room itself, that had two washers and two dryers.

What we needed to have, in our house, for our home and our family to function properly, posed as a distraction from what our house had to offer a new family. The house itself stripped clean to the most simple form, offered a blank canvas for a new family to paint their vision of a home on, yet our home still trying to function within the house only offered distraction. Simplicity sells!

The more I ignored it, the more I fought it, the worse it became. I didn't want simple, unless it came from a wine glass (but even then it would just be a glass because I didn't want to drink to where I couldn't function, or got a headache, or fell asleep … I didn't have time for all that, nor did I want to become an alcoholic).

What I was dealing with was hard, and to slap a smiley face cross sticker on it, wouldn't do *my* hard any justice. I wanted to be hurt, I wanted to be annoyed, I wanted to be angry, I wanted to be sad, and frankly, I wanted people to feel sorry for me.

Talking about my hard with others allowed me to experience a twisted dopamine high. Even though I was mad, sad, and miserable, having people empathize with me made me feel less lonely (crazy how a mom of six can feel lonely when she is rarely ever alone! Loneliness, for me, was more of an inner isolation than outer).

I know you may be thinking there is nothing wrong with wanting to feel like you are not alone. Although on a surface level, that may be true, the problem is, I wasn't dealing with the true issue that was causing my depression. I wasn't the victim of Alzheimer's; my dad was. Yet, I was letting this disease eat away pieces of me, too. I was hurt, I wanted to feel better, but I didn't want to look within myself, that would just be more hard … and I was tired of all the hard.

My partner, Emily, would always tell me how after her dad died, she drank her feelings away. She spent her time, money, and energy in substance abuse to not deal with her hard. I knew I didn't want to go down that rabbit hole.

I had witnessed the devastating effects on both Emily and my brother, so I threw myself in the opposite direction, and unknowingly found myself in another rabbit hole. This hole would prove much darker than I thought possible; this hole that would consume thousands of dollars, hundreds of hours, and much of my energy. I fell into the rabbit hole of self-help.

CHAPTER ELEVEN

The Storm

The Lord is close to the brokenhearted and saves those who are crushed in spirit.

—Psalm 34:18 NIV

The self-help (a.k.a. personal growth or self-improvement) industry is projected to reach $13 billion by 2022.[11] More and more people are eager to fix their conditions and circumstances with online coaching, programs, masterminds, courses, retreats, motivational seminars, apps, and even monthly subscription boxes for all your motivational needs!

I was hooked.

Having had such a positive experience with my John Maxwell program years prior, I wanted to tap into that joy once again. I paid for every single item in the list above, except for the monthly box of motivation, although I sure did follow the maker of the box on Instagram to get my fix.

I was sitting in the car rider line the week after my dad died, not thinking about anything of consequence, but rather I was enjoying the quiet. The car rider line was a coveted place of solace for me.

The littles were at home with a babysitter and, on a few days out of the week, I would leave work to be able to pick up the big boys from school. I learned to watch their faces as they came out of school. I could instantly tell if they'd had a good or bad day just by how they would carry themselves when walking to the car.

I loved the little conversations we had on the way home. However, during this particular season what I looked forward to most was the thirty minutes of waiting in line ... in silence. When the quads were born, our house not only multiplied in the number of people, but it exponentially multiplied in noise level.

On this particular day, however, my silence was interrupted by a divine awakening. God spoke to me and said, "Beloved, get ready for more! Your platform is being established, your story is being crafted from the lessons you are learning. Your father is my precious child and I want you to help others live into their potential by helping them manifest their inspired minds."

Although I did not hear those words with my ears, I heard them with my heart. After looking around in a hesitant manner, I Googled "manifest." That is not a word I use regularly and was a bit unclear of the meaning (confirming my belief that the words were from God).

Manifest: to make evidence of.

Okay ... so I am being called to help others live into their potential by helping someone live in evidence of their inspired mind?

Just as I began to Google "inspired," the car rider line began to move. I set my phone down and began thinking. I had come up with the tagline "Be Inspired" for my salon company over five years prior to this moment.

Two years after that, when the westside salon opened, Emily, Jo, and I all discussed what "Be Inspired" meant for our company. Emily, in solid Emily fashion, Googled it (which is where I learned to do so for *manifest*).

We settled on the definition for *Inspired* that meant "of extraordinary quality." We wanted everything from our systems, to our culture, to our education to be "of extraordinary quality." But how was this definition to play into this new calling? Once the boys were in the car, my thoughts escaped me and I focused on my kids. It wasn't until a few days later that God confirmed the actual meaning he desired me to focus on.

I was home folding laundry and, instead of listening to music per my usual routine, I decided to listen to a podcast. I had a stirring hunger for knowledge and, typically, to satiate that hunger I listen to *John Maxwell Leadership Podcast*, Dean Graziosi's *Millionaire Success Habits*, or *Living Proof* with Beth Moore, but for some reason, I searched out *The Tony Robbins Podcast and* picked a random episode.

A few minutes in, Tony gave the Greek definition for *inspired* as being "in-spirit" or "God-breathed." He carried on with his original point, but I stayed there. Stunned.

I went and grabbed my phone, opened it to Notes, and wrote that little gem down. The Holy Spirit was rejoicing within me … that was it! God was calling me to help others live into their potential by manifesting their inspired minds.

I was to help others use their minds to make evidence of the God-breathed idea put into their lives. Having lost my dad to Alzheimer's, watching him lose control over his thoughts, God was calling me to help others make the most of the ideas God gives them, while their minds are still able.

Once again, God would redeem past pain and turn it into present power.

In a genuine effort of obedience, I leaned way in. So far in, I lost my footing. As I fell into the metaphorical rabbit hole, the walls around me grew darker and seemed to be closing in. I would reach to grab anything for support, anything to slow the fall, anything to offer light, only to have it slip through my fingers.

When I started focusing on what the world was telling me I needed to do ... take courses on how to build a funnel, build a new website, create courses, create Facebook groups, accelerate my business online, grow my Instagram, become an affiliate marketer, grow my email list, learn how to advertise using Pinterest, get rich in your niche, create a money-making blog, start a podcast, create automated email campaigns, and launch programs ... I lost sight of what God had called me to do. I was desperate to find the world's step-by-step process to achieving a divine order.

For each process, in which I invested my time and money, my knowledge of that process expanded. It also revealed other processes I needed to be investing in to get the results I wanted. It was a never-ending cycle and I just kept spinning.

None of what I invested in was bad, wrong, misleading, or corrupt; however, my placing these courses, programs, and processes over my seeking first the kingdom of God led me astray. Out of the dozen-plus self-help strategies I invested in, I only completed one!

I would be on fire to start, I would take massive action, I would implement everything I was learning. Then I would be missing an element needed for success, and instead of finishing the program, I would shift gears and invest in a new program that was all about that particular missing element.

Because I was starting all the things, yet finishing none of the things, I was unfulfilled, mentally exhausted, spiritually weakened, emotionally frustrated, and sickened by the amount of debt I had created. I wanted to add value to people. I wanted to make a massive impact while making an income, yet neither one was happening.

Looking back, I see it all so clearly; but, when I was in the middle of it, I was able to justify each decision and each purchase. I mean, "You have to spend money to make money," or "Riches are in the niches," or "You have to have an abundance mindset over a scarcity mindset," or "With great risk comes great reward," or "You have to invest to get a return on your investment." None of these sayings are necessarily wrong or bad, but I had used them to justify spending money I did not have, putting my family and my company in a vulnerable position, and that was reckless of me.

I wasn't even consciously aware of how reckless it was until I was willing to forgo taking my big boys to Harry Potter World for their birthdays so that I could attend a mastermind in Arkansas.

I wanted to first make an impact, but I also wanted to make an income, not just to be able to retire my mom and my husband, but also to be able to afford the lives we were trying to build.

We wanted to travel, having adventure experiences with our kids. Matt and I love food and going on a culinary journey. Trying new places and new tastes together make for some of our favorite dates!

The sheer cost of having six kids is beyond what we ever imagined ... especially when sickness comes through the house bringing doctor's visits, prescription costs, etc.

We should have purchased stock in Tylenol®, Lysol®, and Pedialyte®. We required two washers, two dryers, two ovens, and two dishwashers.

Matt and I have always said we don't need to be financially sitting pretty, we just want to be able to buy our kids new clothes and shoes when they outgrow them within a few months' time.

I would love to shop more for the healthy and organic foods that better care for our bodies. I want to get all the foods we need at the grocery store without breaking into a cold sweat at the checkout line because I have gone over our budget.

We want to be able to go on vacation without having saved a whole year to fund it. How nice would it be, and how much would it mean to our marriage, to be able to go on more than one date night every few months?

These things may seem trivial, but they matter to us.

* * *

After the quads' first birthday, Matt won an all-expenses-paid trip to Hawaii through his company. We were beyond ecstatic. Neither of us had ever been to Hawaii, and we had not had a trip alone together in over two years.

The first year of parenting six was a complete whirlwind— kids and kids' stuff everywhere! We lived in a sleepless haze surrounded by a never-ending mountain of dishes and laundry.

We dealt with the constant guilt of feeling inadequate as attentive parents to our big boys. We were so consumed in survival mode that our time together consisted of brief kisses on our way to and from the house and high fives when we had a great teamwork moment.

Every day, I fell more in love with Matt, and my gratitude for my partner grew even deeper. I thought our marriage was at a high point because of all that we were accomplishing together. I didn't realize those feelings were not mutual.

Hawaii was as beautiful as I had imagined it to be. The ocean, the cliffs, the lush landscapes. As amazing as they were, they came in second to the fresh fruits, fish, and coffee we enjoyed daily. We spent the first day at the beach allowing the sun to revive our tired bodies.

Matt decided to walk the shoreline looking for shells to take back to the big boys. The waves were over six feet tall that afternoon and the shoreline was not smooth sand, but boulders and volcanic rocks. Matt was already teetering atop a boulder when he was taken out by a wave. I watched him go down and giggled to myself at the sight of his 6'4" slender body flailing through the air.

Once I saw him surface, I closed my eyes, smiling, and drifted asleep. Moments later, I heard him grunting as he approached our cabana. Through squinted eyes, I saw him limping towards me.

He sat down and lifted his foot to show me his mangled toe that was beginning to turn red. He said the pain was so excruciating, it was making him nauseated.

I peered at him over my sunglasses and said, "I'm so sorry your stubbed toe hurts, I birthed four babies at once." Granted, that wasn't the most loving response, but Matt tends to be a bit of a hypochondriac.

An hour or so later, I woke up to see him passed out. When I looked down at his toe, I cringed to see it had turned a deep maroon and tripled its usual size. Clearly, he was due some sympathy. I used the plastic bag lining the ice bucket with its remaining cubes to create an ice pack.

I elevated his foot with a towel and placed the impromptu compress on his toe, waking him up in the process. Later that night, we laughed about the great start to our vacation. Then, we enjoyed some incredible food and some much-needed intimate time together.

The next day, we were scheduled to do the Jurassic Park™ ATV tour around the island. Matt's toe was so swollen he couldn't fit his foot into his shoe.

We were standing at the bus waiting to go on the tour when the director told us Matt would not be able to go on the excursion without wearing closed-toe shoes.

I quickly ran back to our room and grabbed his tennis shoes, making a quick stop to go to the bathroom while I was there.

Great! Not only did Matt have a broken toe, but I had just started my period.

As I ran back to the bus, I prayed that God would have mercy on the rest of our vacation. This time away was supposed to be excursions, culinary ventures, and all the love-making we had been missing out on.

Instead, we encountered Broken Toe Beach and an uninvited Aunt Flo. We did our best to make the most of the remainder of our vacation, reminding ourselves of how thankful we were to have a FREE trip to Hawaii, but something felt off. Perhaps it was because we had built up this vacation so much in our minds before we left, that when our plans didn't go as expected, we felt gypped.

Once we returned home, we had a hard time getting back into our routine. We were going through all the right motions, but getting all the wrong results. I hadn't realized how robotic I had become (not only with my mommy duties but also with my way of being) until I was taken out of it for a week.

One evening, after all the kids had gone down for the night, I sat on our bed, folding laundry. Matt walked in and sat at the foot of the bed, facing away from me.

"I'm unhappy in our marriage," he muttered. I sat in silence, confused at what he had just said. He continued, "I thought Hawaii would help us re-connect, but the whole trip just felt 'off.'"

I had to force myself to break the silence. "So … what does that mean? Are you wanting to be done?" More silence.

"What changed?" I asked. "I thought we were doing great. I mean, I know it has been really hard and taxing, but I thought we were doing 'the hard' pretty well together."

His only response was staring at the floor, so I kept going.

"I need you to tell me more. What does you being 'unhappy in our marriage' mean for us? Are you saying you want to be done?"

As much as I wanted to ask him if he wanted a divorce, I had always deeply believed that you don't mention the word "divorce" until you were willing to accept what all that meant. And at that moment, I was not.

Finally, he responded.

"I mean … I'm not going to leave you and our family … I'm not a quitter."

"You aren't a quitter? I don't want you to be in this marriage because 'you aren't a quitter!' How about, I don't want to leave because I love you and this family we created together? Not because you are not a quitter!" I could feel the heat rising into my ears.

"Well … no … that's not what I meant. I just don't feel like we connect anymore. This has been really hard."

"What … What has been really hard?" I interrupted.

"This ... All of this!" He motioned his arms in large circles as he loudly continued. "I only ever wanted one child and now I have six. You were going to be a stay-at-home mom and now you have multiple companies that are drowning us in debt. We have no time together. We are just now getting to sleep through the night! And to be honest, I'm jealous that our kids get all your time and energy and I get what's left. And we know that's not much."

I couldn't control the tears welling up. My mind was racing.

What in the world did he expect of me? I was trying my best, and once again I had fallen short.

He is my husband and partner. We are supposed to be in this together. He thinks he has it hard? Try being the f*'king mommy ... that's what's hard.

The thoughts swarmed and my emotions ran hot. I knew if I spoke, I would do more harm than good. I knew if I tried to respond, it would be a reaction in disguise.

After several long minutes, he continued. "I'm not going to leave. I don't want to leave. I love our family, but I'm not happy."

And with one word, he lit the dynamite I had desperately been trying to hide.

"Not HAPPY? Who said life was about being happy? Happy is an illusion! If you are basing your happiness on other people or circumstances, you will never be truly happy. God calls us to be joyful, not happy. You think I'm HAPPY all the time? You think I ENJOY how hard this all is? You think this is what I planned for my life? You think raising six kids, running multiple businesses, and being a 'good' wife is all giggles and rainbows? It is f**king hard!

"And when I need you the most ... when we need to be a strong team, you are 'unhappy'? Nine out of ten showers are spent with me crying on the shower floor. It is the ONLY time I get to myself. Everybody ALWAYS needs me for something. I can't even go to the bathroom without being interrupted. If it's not the kids, it's my employees, if it's not my employees, it's you ... I am NEEDED all day, every day! HAPPY? Do you think all this is my 'happy'?"

Without hesitation he fired back: "Then quit! If your job no longer makes you happy ... quit. If you are so miserable at home ... leave, I know that's what you have always wanted."

All of a sudden I could see again. My rage was fading and I saw this argument for what it was.

For our entire marriage, Matt had struggled with insecurity. Even in the beginning, with every tiny fight, he would ask if I was going to leave him. Matt's parents had divorced when he was in his early twenties. Some wounds run so deep that simply moving on doesn't heal them properly.

Still shaking, I approached where he was sitting.

Standing in front of him, I placed my hands gently around his face: "I love you! I have never wanted and do not want to leave you. I meant what I said in our vows 'for better or worse.' We are in the 'worse' right now."

Now, sitting on his lap, I continued, "Anytime things get hard, you push me away. I don't know, maybe you are trying to protect yourself. But it feels like you want to push me away so that I will leave, and you can say 'I told you so.' Look at me! I'm not going anywhere. I don't want anyone else. This life we have created together may be hard, really, really hard ... but we can do hard ... together.

"'Who God joins together, let no man tear apart,' and you are

included in that. I know your parents got divorced, but we are not your parents. My dad meant what he said to you when you asked for my hand in marriage: 'no take-backs!'"

We both laughed.

"I need you to understand, Matt. I am not living for the next thing that will make me happy. I am living this life to experience all the joy that God has designed it for. That includes you, and our kids, and my company, and my family. Joy is found in his perfect love lived out in our daily lives.

"I want my life to reflect all who he is. Do I suck at it sometimes? Of course I do! He loves me anyway. I know that no matter what we encounter, when we face it together, we are better. We may not always do it well, but it will still be better."

I would love to say that with those words and the love-making that followed, we were all good. But the truth is, I was hurt. For the next several months, I walked on eggshells, afraid that any little argument would destroy our fragile marriage. I had been praying so hard for God to fix Matt, so he wouldn't feel so insecure, until one day, my prayers shifted.

"God, I can't change my husband. You love him just as much as you love me. There is no right or wrong here. He is hurt, I am hurt, and we need to be healed. Lord, change me. Show me what I can do to fix me. If he is who he is forevermore, help me to grow. Help me to be who he needs me to be. Who YOU designed me to be, for him. Help us to seek you first. Show us the way to live out our marriage in the way you have created it to be. Amen."

Slowly, God began mending my brokenness. Slowly, God softened Matt's heart and he allowed himself to be more vulnerable. Knowing that Matt had some deep unresolved trust issues, I did not need to be the one giving him advice or suggestions, so we met with a counselor.

My place, during this time, was to be supportive, encouraging, and truthful about my feelings. I made a promise to myself that no matter what the counselor said, I would never chime back with an "I told you so." I did not have to be right; we had to get it right.

✻ ✻ ✻

Years later, Matt and I are still working on our marriage.

We fall back into old habits and insecurities when we are under stress; however, now we are able to get each other back out of it much easier. We have learned that making time to enjoy *us* is vital to the success of our marriage.

Before we were a family, we were a *we*. And before the *we*, there was *me*.

This journey of self-help had been repressed for years. Why did it take a HUGE life event to make me want to take care of myself? My first real experience of self-help was when I was pregnant with quadruplets and I joined the John Maxwell Team.

The next would be after my dad died.

I guess that behavior can be typical of most moms. We eat last. Typical? Maybe, but this round mutated quickly from growing into my best self, to be able to best serve others, to making money.

When my ambition for making income replaced my *why* behind making the income, I knew I had faltered. So naturally, in my self-help obsession and new awareness, what did I do? I reached out to a successful social media influencer I had been following.

This particular influencer was not like other influencers on social media. Rachel was more about being honest, raw, and genuine. She cares more about being influential in someone's life than trying to influence them to buy a particular product.

Rachel was opening a small group, an online mastermind, about how to put on a profitable speaking event. I had been a speaker for high school students before and loved every minute of it.

Maybe investing in Rachel's mastermind would give me the skills I needed to host my first event. I could help a lot of people and make enough money to pay off the credit card debt I had accumulated by trying to reach my audience through every other platform. It made perfect sense.

However, when I reached out to Rachel and vaguely over-viewed what I had invested in thus far, I fully expected her to tell me I was a perfect candidate for her mastermind. I just knew she would be able to get me where I needed to go and to achieve what I was looking for.

Thankfully, she did not. Rachel, being the amazing, kind, and honest person she is, called me on my crap. In a few brief Instagram messages, she called me out for being a course junkie!

She told me I was doing all the right things but needed the patience to see them work. She didn't try to sell me her mastermind; she didn't try to sell me her coaching. She simply saw how to best serve me, and that was by telling me the ugly truth.

I instantly knew she was right, yet I was supposed to take massive action. That's what successful entrepreneurs do, right? I had an abundance mindset. I was going to make a difference! I just needed my big break.

After all, this was God's idea! He brought me to it, therefore he will bring me through it. And although that is 100% true, God doesn't do the *easy* way out. He loves us too much to uproot us from the trenches and place us on the mountain top.

Where is the growth in our faith there? God never promises an easy life, in fact, he promises the contrary. 2 Corinthians 4:8-10 (NIV) says: "We are hard-pressed on every side, but not crushed; perplexed, but not in despair; persecuted, but not abandoned; struck down, but not destroyed. We always carry around in our body the death of Jesus, so that the life of Jesus may also be revealed in our body." So even though we go through crushing despair or persecution, we are never alone. The way out has already been provided.

I learned the hard way that it takes patience and practice to correct the lies we tell ourselves and courage to replace them with truth.

Several times after my reality check with Rachel, I would still be tempted to do more, to be more, to invest in more! That is how the enemy works. I wasn't being tempted in ways that were obviously harmful to me and my relationship with the Lord, no no, the enemy is much more clever than that. He discovered what was already working and made it more accessible to me.

Spiritual warfare is real. The devil is a schemer. He comes to kill, steal, and destroy and he rarely announces himself (John 10:10 NIV).

Just as God sends people and opportunities into your life to help you grow in your faith, the enemy does the same, except his mission is to diminish your faith and drive a divide between you and God.

Scripture tells us to "Put on the full armor of God, so that you can take your stand against the devil's schemes. For our struggle is not against flesh and blood, but against the rulers, against the authorities, against the powers of this dark world and against the spiritual forces of evil in the heavenly realms." Ephesians 6:11-12 (NIV)

So next time you think you don't have enough value for the enemy to pursue you, think again! You are a precious child of God and are therefore more valuable than wealth, stature, fame, or position. I know I can stand firm on this foundation of truth, but that doesn't mean my legs don't get wobbly.

CHAPTER TWELVE

The Hurricane

*Be strong and immovable. Always work enthusiastically for
the Lord, for you know that nothing you do
for the Lord is ever useless.*

—1 Corinthians 15:58 NLT

Life was beginning to look up ... ish. I had realized the
error of my self-help ways. Although I was still committed to living into my best self, I had promised myself
that I would not purchase another course, mastermind, program, or seminar until I was able to pay down some debt.

The salon was beginning to turn a profit. We were growing
both in numbers and our team's size. We were excited to
invest in the education and training of four of our team
members by sending them to Las Vegas for four days. Emily
and Jo tried to talk me out of paying for our employees'
tickets, but I refused to concede.

My dad always believed in doing what was right for his employees (he was a Chick-fil-A operator for 18 years). He would
always go above and beyond to show his team that they were
loved and appreciated, inviting them to family BBQ or over
to play basketball, helping to pay a bill or put gas in someone's car.

The "troubled teen" always found their place in my dad's store. His heart was always bigger than his wallet. I followed closely in my dad's footsteps. I wanted to honor my dad's memory by investing in my people as he did his.

Emily and Jo had valid points that our employees needed to have a little skin in the game. They needed to invest some of their personal money to go on this trip to show they were just as committed to growing their skills and education as we were.

Although I fully understood their point, I thought of all the times I had prayed for help. If I had someone believe in me enough to invest their money in our company, I wouldn't have to borrow from the bank.

I wanted to be able to give to someone, or rather four some-ones, what I had only dreamed someone would believe in me enough to do. I convinced my partners that we needed to fully invest in our people.

We could put their tickets on our company's American Express Card®. Doing so would allow us the grace needed to not take the large financial hit at one time.

Emily and I were set to go with our four team members to Vegas. I had never been to this advanced training and was excited to have the opportunity to learn from some of the best in the country.

Sadly, my excitement was short-lived. Although he agreed, Matt was extremely uncomfortable with me going to Vegas. He tried his best to be fully on board, but he simply wasn't. The strain it was already putting on our marriage was not worth what I would learn in Vegas. Emily was willing to continue on as chaperone and owner, learning for both of us.

Months after their return from Vegas, we saw a large spike

in our sales. The advanced education really paid off for these ladies. They not only learned much, but they were also applying what they learned, and that is when you see results. Results indeed! Our team continued to grow and the financial debt noose began to feel looser.

Seeing how well our salon was doing, Emily agreed to accompany me in my new side hustle. I had invested so much time, money, and energy into all my self-help courses and training, that I felt it was the perfect time to apply all I had learned. The way I figured it, the more I was able to impact others, the more income I could make.

The more income I made, the faster I could pay off all my personal and salon debt. Once all the salon debt was paid off, we owners could start drawing a significant distribution check.

Win, win, win!

The three of us desperately needed to be making money from our company. I was feeling the financial strain of six kids, the remaining Eastside debt, and training debt. Emily had welcomed her second baby. Jo had become an insta-parent (and I don't mean Instagram, I mean instant).

* * *

Nine months prior, we sat in the office praying that Jo would be able to adopt or foster a specific baby that was currently in utero. The situation surrounding this precious forming child was complicated to say the least.

As the months passed, Jo never heard anything more about the baby or the baby's mother. We all had assumed the worst, that the mom had relapsed or had an abortion.

Shortly after Christmas, Jo received a phone call. The baby had just been born, and she needed to come and pick him up if she wanted him.

Two days later, I received a phone call. Jo was driving up my street and frantically asked me to meet her in my driveway. I raced outside just as she was getting out of the car. She ran to me shaking with tears streaming down her face.

Gasping for breath between sobs, she asked me to look in her back seat.

The past year had been especially hard for Jo. After two failed engagements, she believed she had found the right man for her. He was loving and attentive. He had a good head on his shoulders. He was an established professional. He was supportive and encouraging of her advancing her career. He was "the one." Or so we all believed. Everything listed above was a lie. The details of her story are captivating, but it is her story to tell.

Approaching her car, all I could think about was where my shovel was. I just knew her ex had come after her and in self-defense she murdered him. Now she was scared and in my driveway. It was go-time. I had to force myself to swallow as I opened the back door.

Praise Jesus! The body in the back seat was an infant!

Jo was a mom.

No planning, no nesting, no nothing. She picked up a car seat on the way to the hospital, without a single hesitation that this baby would be hers.

She felt completely inadequate to assume the role, but she knew God had called her to this moment and she was not about to let fear keep her from walking in obedience.

* * *

We were young, first-time business owners trying our best to keep our individual worlds spinning while growing and supporting all those who worked with us and our guests.

Additional income would have been the floating device needed as we were all exhausted from treading water. Since this new company, Sorella Inspired, would not be brick and mortar, but rather online, we would not need to go to the bank for a loan.

Emily was fully gifted in the area of computers and I was the visionary. I would create the content and she would get it out there.

Such a simple plan, what could go wrong?

All the things. All the things could and did go wrong.

We had decided to strike while the iron was hot.

While the salon was seeing more money, we decided to go ahead and trademark our salon name, the ll's from our logo, and The Inspired Life. I would also solely open a tertiary company, Sorella Enterprises, to be the umbrella for all the companies that would follow in the upcoming years. Our five-year plan included opening a cosmetology school and another Sorella Suites location.

The world was our oyster and we were ready to dump hot sauce all over it!

Trademarking involves attorneys and fees. Although Emily did much of the work herself, we still had to purchase a domain for our new website. We created The Inspired Life Journal. Printing, marketing, and selling the journals all required funds. Our American Express was earning a lot of miles.

Because Sorella Suites was holding steady with its renters, and Sorella Hair Studio was showing profit, I was able to make any and all payments owed. That is until we experienced our first mass exodus.

Four of our employees (including two we had invested in for Vegas) and a suite renter got together and decided to go open their own salon. Under normal circumstances, I would have been saddened by this news, but the amount of lying that went into protecting their secret created a whole new level of hurt and betrayal.

From the moment I interview someone to come work for us, I tell her how much I despise lying. Every decision will come with a consequence. Lying to me only makes the consequence more difficult.

A few months prior, Emily, Jo, and I felt our team was off. We had never had a team so large. We had never had so much on our individual plates. We were in new territory. After staff meetings and individual meetings asking our team for their participation in helping us get this right, we chalked up our unsettled feeling to growing pains.

Since the quads started sleeping through the night, I never had trouble sleeping. I was so flipping tired by the end of the day, my body and mind embraced sleep like a long-lost friend. During the day my mind would easily get swayed into a state of worry, but at night I laid my worries down knowing the Bible verse "If God is for us, who can be against us?" (Romans 8:31 NIV) and would quickly fall asleep. Even though we agreed our feelings were just feelings, I knew deep down, a ball was about to drop, and I feared I would be the one doing the dropping. For the first time in a long time, I wrestled with sleep.

I always thought the "If God was for me, who can be against me" verse meant that because I was a believer and was living, for all intents and purposes, a right and integrous life, that no one would come against me.

Turns out, that is not at all what that verse means.

Scripture tells us "no weapon formed against you shall prosper" in Isaiah 54:17 (NKJV), but it doesn't say no weapon will be formed!

I confronted the ringleader of the exodus group, and asked her to come to me, with her integrity intact, and tell me what was going on.

The condensation growing on our water glasses paled in comparison to the amount of sweat being produced from her palms.

Both Emily and Jo traded glances at each other and back to me, silently begging for me to interrupt the silence. I sat tall and calm, staring into her wandering eyes.

After shifting in her seat and fidgeting with her bracelets, she fumbled for words as she hesitantly told me a version of what was happening. I felt so conflicted.

Part of me wanted to hug and congratulate her for living into her dreams, while another part of me wanted to vomit for letting my guard down. Just a month prior I had asked her to meet with me outside of the salon. I pleaded with her to share any information she might know as to why our team felt so off.

I looked directly into her eyes and asked her if she had my back ... to which she responded, "Yes."

Inadvertently lying to me is bad and has its own consequences, but straight-faced lying to me is not tolerable.

At the end of our meeting, we had agreed to let them work out a notice. That night, I went home and was sick to my stomach. I started thinking back to all the conversations I had had with those who were leaving and my heart began to break.

* * *

How had I created so much fear within my team that not one of them felt secure enough to come have an honest conversation with me?

I spent years investing my time, energy, and money into growing these women ... and for what?

Did they not care about all the sacrifices I had made to keep their professional world spinning?

Sure, it was great they grew in their skills enough to go out on their own, but that was not what was bothering me. I was happy for their professional growth, but I was devastated that after all this time, not one of them trusted who I was enough to come to me in truth.

If I couldn't grow people I worked with daily, people I saw face to face, people I shared my life with, how would I ever be able to grow people that found me online? I am 34 years old, have multiple businesses, a slew of kids, a fragile marriage, and apparently no freaking clue what I'm doing! As my world came crashing down, sleep was nowhere to be found.

* * *

Sometimes you need a sleepless night to finally wake up! I came into work the next day, tired, sickened, but assured. I knew I could no longer work with people who could lie to me so easily. They were asked to leave that afternoon.

Our company's revenue was cut in half. We were no longer hitting the numbers needed to pay all our bills. Emily, Jo, and I felt betrayed. We questioned if our company was Humpty Dumpty.

After experiencing a great fall, completely shattered, would we be able to put it back together again? We didn't know how to move forward or who we could trust. If we made a decision someone didn't like, would they leave too? Did the employees who remained secretly steal client information to give to those who had left?

Our minds were swarming with all the possible conspiracy theories. None of which helped us heal or move forward. We knew we were too hurt to authentically lead from our hearts anymore, yet we also knew leading from a place of fear served no one.

Out of sheer desperation and emotional exhaustion, we discussed various exit strategies. Selling a non-profitable business was not a viable option. Switching our staff from employees to renters would have worked had we not been carrying such a heavy debt load. After meeting with a bankruptcy attorney we realized carrying on as before was our only viable option. We decided to take emotion out of it and stick to the facts:

Fact 1: Our income was cut in half.

Fact 2: We did not have enough stylists to service our growing guest count.

Fact 3: Emily and I were not licensed to do the hair.

We laid it all out and began to work the problem. We had grown our company before. We knew which systems worked and which didn't.

Emily, Jo, and I agreed that we would be strictly solution-minded when at work, and if we needed to vent our emotions we did it out of the salon. We could not afford to bring our insecurities and fears into the building but had to keep an open, honest line of communication among the three of us.

The fear wasn't gone. I faced it every morning as I logged into our bank account or had to pay the bills or pay our taxes. No, the fear and the pain were ever-present, but just because I felt paralyzed by the fear, it did not excuse inaction.

Whether I wanted to face our debt or not, it was there, glaring at me in red. I had to put my big-girl panties on and deal with it. I couldn't *believe* my way out of it. Noah had to BUILD the ark! Yes, faith was required, but he had to pick up the hammer and get to work!

My personal life was put on hold for the entire month of June. I was on autopilot for everything that wasn't Sorella Hair Studio. My first Father's Day without my dad was approaching and, although I set aside that one day to be out of the salon to spend time with my mom, brother, and sister and have much needed time to grieve, not a single tear was shed. Despite all the facts, the truth was I was numb.

Have you heard the saying "God won't give you more than you can handle"? I learned that statement is false. God will 100% give you more than you can handle, or at least allow you to experience more than you can handle because we live in a fallen world.

You know what he won't do though? He won't leave you there alone. He won't turn a blind eye. He won't choose to help someone else over you. He won't stay silent when you ask him to speak. He won't deny you your request for his wisdom. He won't refuse you his peace that passes all understanding. He won't dismiss your cries for help because you are "too far gone."

God will give you more than you can handle, but he will never give you more than the two of you can handle together! Being a believer doesn't mean you won't face challenges that break you down; however, when you endure, you learn that God allows you to be broken in order to rebuild you stronger than before.

Putting the pieces back together, I learned that I cannot pour into those who feel they are already full. I cannot share wisdom with those who already know all there is to know. I cannot lead those who are unwilling to follow. I cannot invest in people who are unwilling to invest in themselves. I cannot help those who are unwilling to see error in their actions.

I can, however, choose to focus on those whom God is placing in my path. I can choose not to let the hurt I feel hurt others. I can choose to see the light through the darkness. I can choose to share the love and inspiration that God has graciously shown me.

CHAPTER THIRTEEN

The Water Walker

*Do not conform to the pattern of this world, but be
transformed by the renewing of your mind. Then you will
be able to test and approve what God's will is—
his good, pleasing and perfect will.*

—Romans 12:2 NIV

I was always hesitant to pray for God's will to be done in
my life. I had heard all these miraculous stories of overwhelming, tragic, or catastrophic events or circumstances that nearly destroyed a person's life.

In these compelling stories, the sufferer would have expo-
nential transformation and healing by clinging to God for his
strength and mercy. These stories were inspirational and
moving. As much as I desired to inspire and impact others, I
feared if I prayed for God's will in my life, I would be put
through the fire.

My life's storms, thus far, had tested and broken me in ways
I never fathomed; yet, I couldn't help but think my experiences were minimal compared to what others have had to
endure. What would walking through fire look like in my life?

Tony Robbins is a famous author, philanthropist, and life

coach. He holds seminars all around the world helping people discover their personal power. In one of his seminars, he has the audience literally walk through fire via hot coals.

Tony says, "We are trained, almost innately, to be scared of fire and to keep away from it. That is why walking through a pathway of fire is a powerful expression of moving beyond one's fears."[12] I always felt encouraged by this sentiment; yet, in hearing of all the thousands of "firewalkers," I have only ever heard of one inspired leader who walked on water.

In the book of Matthew, we learn the story:

Shortly before dawn Jesus went out to them, walking on the lake. When the disciples saw him walking on the lake, they were terrified. "It's a ghost," they said, and cried out in fear.

But Jesus immediately said to them: "Take courage! It is I. Don't be afraid."

"Lord, if it's you," Peter replied, "tell me to come to you on the water."

"Come," he said.

Then Peter got down out of the boat, walked on the water and came toward Jesus. But when he saw the wind, he was afraid and, beginning to sink, cried out, "Lord, save me!"

Immediately Jesus reached out his hand and caught him. "You of little faith," he said, "why did you doubt?" Matthew 14:25-31 (NIV).

Firewalkers must quickly get across the coals! If they linger too long they will be burned. In order for Peter to walk on water, he was not asked to move swiftly. He was not warned if he stood still, he would sink. Peter only began to sink when he took his eyes off Jesus and feared the wind's coming.

Perhaps God was teaching me that many can make it through the fire relying on their own strength, the guidance of others, their willingness to disobey their fears; but only those who take courage in the Lord can ever walk on water.

Perhaps it is in the little steps of consistent faith we learn our true power ... the power of God within us.

Perhaps the water we must learn to walk on is made up of our daily struggles, those events that may seem "minimal" but require all the faith that we can muster.

Faith is faith, no matter how small.

Perhaps we must learn that going through the sh*t in life is what is required to create a shiFt in our life. Perhaps manifesting God's strength within us is the only way to transform our trials into testimonies of triumph.

In my business, I had to learn to see the forest through the trees. This concept was hard for me to grasp as I felt as though I was trying to view the forest while running on the ground, getting smacked in the face by various branches.

My "water" was learning the truth behind the pains that most shook my faith. It wasn't the mass exodus I had, it was questioning all the small decisions I had made leading up to their departure.

It wasn't my husband saying he was unhappy in our marriage, it was all the excuses I had made to no longer need to be attentive to him. It wasn't the massive debt I had generated, it was the selfish desire behind it.

It wasn't losing my dad at such a young age to a horribly unfair disease; it was forgiving myself for the consuming regret caused by all the moments I missed with him out of sheer annoyance toward his behavior.

It wasn't the physical torment of my breast implant illness; it was coming to terms with my insecurity that put them there.

It wasn't the physical, emotional, mental, and spiritual pain I endured while carrying quadruplets; it was learning to navigate the foreign territory both within my body and within my loneliness.

Every event in my life, big or small, has called for some degree of faith. Sometimes faith came easier, sometimes not. But faith was required, nonetheless.

If you were to ask me, "What is the worst kind of pain to go through? Physical, spiritual, emotional, or mental?"

I would say, "Whichever kind of pain you are going through right now!"

No matter how your pain compares to another's, it is still pain. Comparison is not only the thief of joy, but it is also the inhibitor of peace and healing.

Once I stopped comparing the midst of my storms to someone else's rainbows, I was able to more clearly see and trust in how God was working it for my good.

Whenever I was engulfed by a current pain, wounds of my past seemed less significant. When I was recovering from the birth of the quads, I was experiencing the most physical pain I had ever had.

The pain was so intense I doubted I would ever experience anything worse. When my dad died, the emotional pain I had was so intense, I doubted if I had or would ever experience anything worse.

The two pains were completely different. One brought life and the other was over the loss of it. No matter which pain you are experiencing, or have just come out of, know that if you have breath in your lungs and a thought in your mind, there is hope.

Surrender the knowledge of how your situation might turn out and start looking up. Only elevation will allow you to see the forest through the trees. The same branches that hit you in the face are still there, but they can no longer reach you!

Keep your eyes on Jesus. Allow yourself to take hold of his promise to give you hope and a future. And place your foot upon the stepping stone forged in preserving faith and left for you in love.

I never dreamed God would transform my pain and the hardest times in my life to reflect joy and perseverance. I never dreamed God would use my trials to create a depth in me that would allow me to better see, love, and serve others. My lack of dreaming bigger proved that God's ways were always higher than my own.

When I finally released my illusion of all that had happened *to* me and replaced it with the truth of all God had done *for* me, I could no longer claim victim, only VICTORY!

You see, God has shown me that the storms will come and the waters will rise, but he is continually showing me how to walk on water!

God is our refuge and strength, a very present help in trouble. Therefore will not we fear, though the earth be removed, and though the mountains be carried into the midst of the sea; though the waters thereof roar and be troubled, though the mountains shake with the swelling thereof.

—Psalm 46:1-3 KJV

AFTERWORD

It took a global pandemic, the permanent closure of my salon company, and filing personal bankruptcy before I acted on my decision to pursue my ideal future—the future in which God promises prosperity and hope.

Every storm, struggle, and hardship that occurred previously was like a guiding light from a burning fire. If only I would have moved when I first saw the light instead of waiting until I felt the heat!

The light taught me lessons and allowed me to learn, but the heat is what caused me to move.

And the truth is, you will remain stuck unless you decide to take action. Because just as Noah had to pick up his hammer to build the ark God had called him to build, so must you pick up your tools to build the future God is calling you into.

I believe just as God is molding you in your journey from point A (who you are now) to point B (who you are called to be), so you are molding your tools.

Each new lesson learned, each obstacle overcome, each struggle surrendered develops a new tool for building your future.

Tools can also be gained in the wisdom shared by someone who has gone before you, in the generosity of helping hands, the care and encouragement of the community, and in the proven instruction of a coach or mentor.

It's funny how driving in circles is maddening, but when life's moments come full circle, there is an element of peace and assurance that everything you endured along the way was worth it.

Learning how to confidently and purposefully live out God's promise has been that full circle moment for me.

You see, the best version of you is 100% still available to you. All the things you have been through are just more tools in your toolbox for building your future. It's not too late, and you do have the time.

HOW TO GET MORE HELP

I f life has you feeling like you are drowning, know this: Learning to rise above challenging circumstances and overwhelming obstacles isn't easy, but it is possible!

I believe God is using every ounce of my past pain for good, as a way to clear the path for another, transforming my stumbling blocks into stepping stones for someone else.

And as I promised all those who asked me "how" I was going to _____ (fill in the blank). When I learned "how" I did it, I would share it.

The ARISE Formula: Five Steps To Elevating Your Mindset will help you:

- Renew Your Mind

- Clarify Your Calling

- Transform Your Life

For more inspiration, life lessons, and all-around good laughs, join the Inspired Life Community Facebook Group at: **www.facebook.com/groups/inspiredlifefreegroup**

If you desire to learn how to "walk on water" in your life, find out how you can work with Julianne here: **www.inspiredlifementor.com/workwithme**

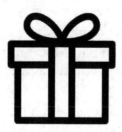

FREE GIFT

Download Julianne's ARISE Formula—Five Steps to Elevating Your Mindset HERE:

www.inspiredlifementor.com/audio-download

OUR JOURNEY

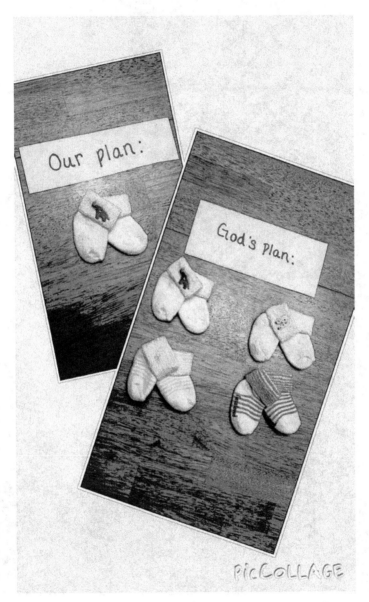

*Our Pregnancy Announcement: Proof God's Ways
Are Always Higher than Our Own!*

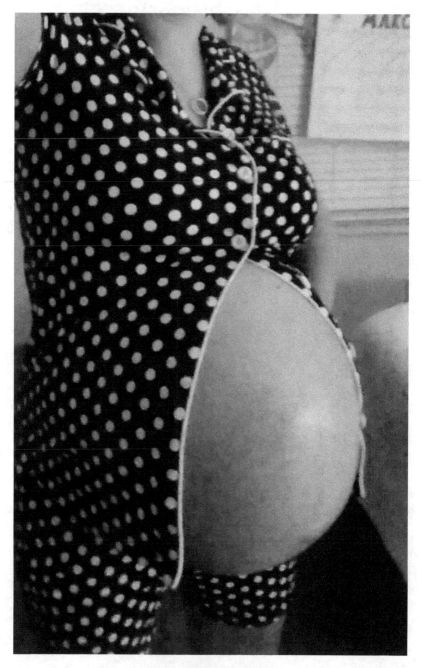

That's One Big Belly

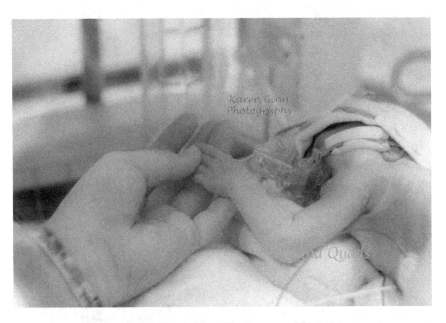

A Long-Awaited First Embrace with Ashton

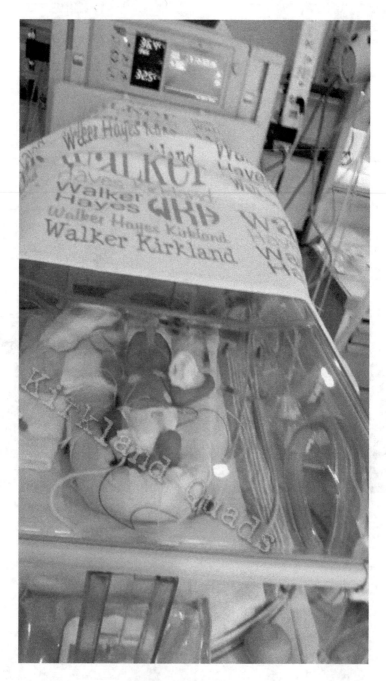

Walker in His Isolette

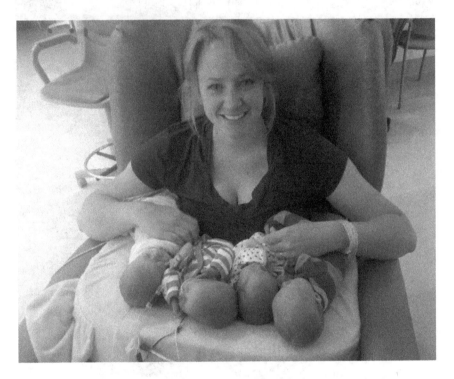

First Time Together Again

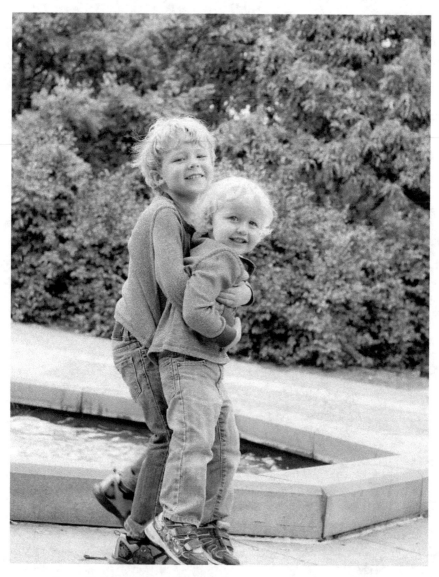

Campbell and Jack Before They Became Outnumbered

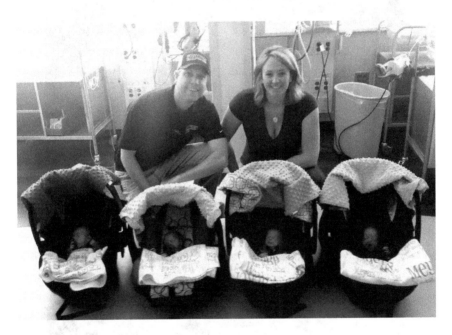

All Going Home on the Same Day!

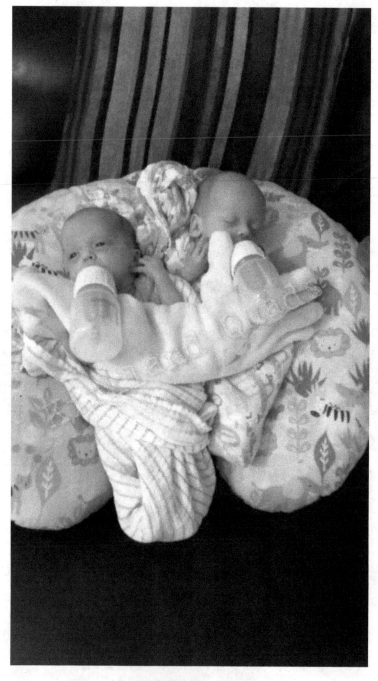

Bottle Propping Success

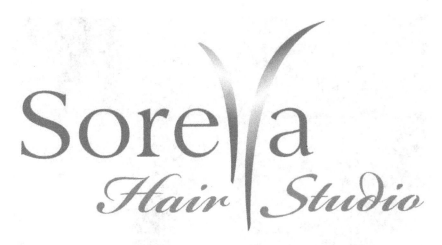

Our First Salon Logo

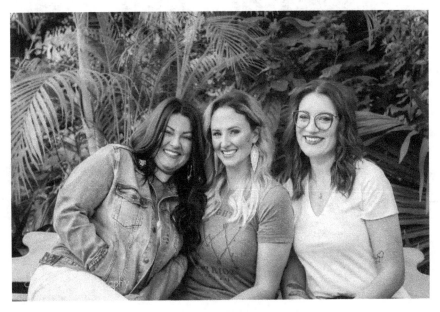

My Partners Jo and Emily

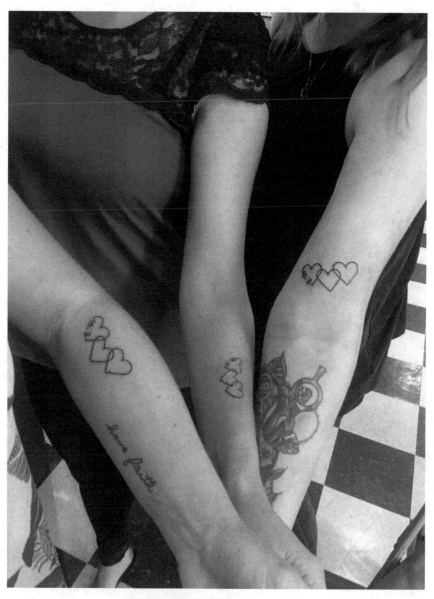

Our Proverbs 16:3 Tattoo

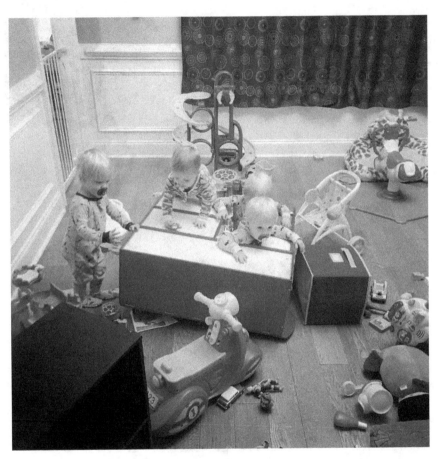

The Most Destructive Force on the Planet ... the QUADNADO!

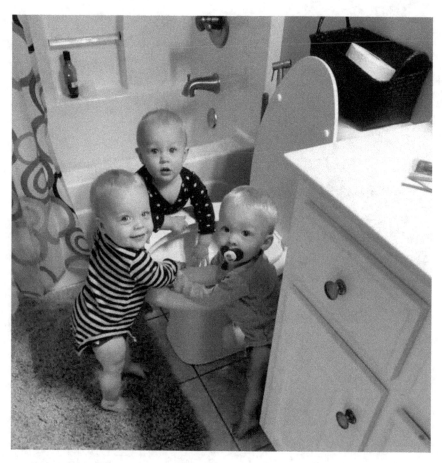

Triple Trouble

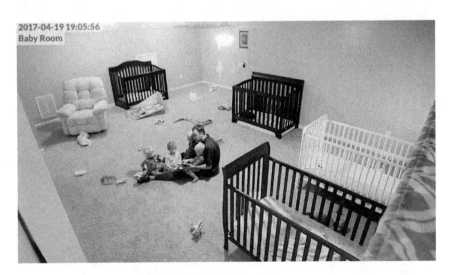

Daddy Time in the Nursery

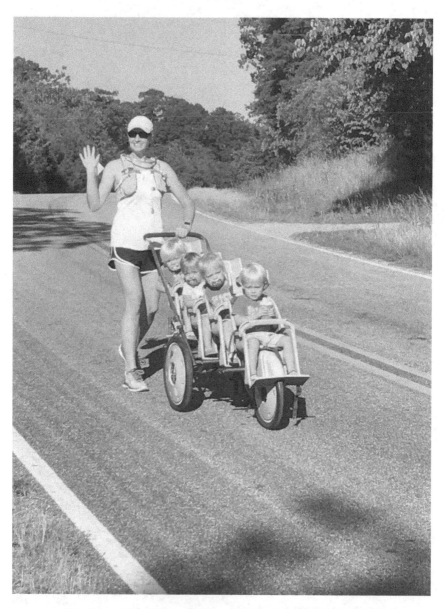

The Quad Stroller — Where Even Running Downhill Feels Like Uphill

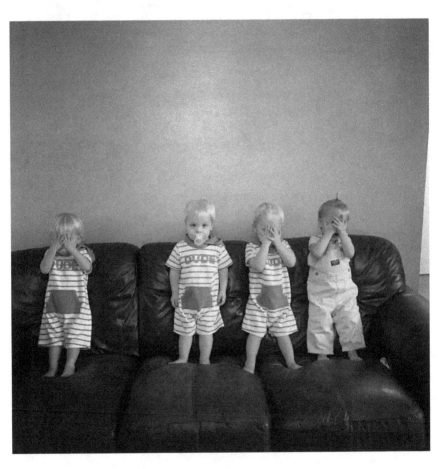

"Who Did It?" — Meyers Did It.

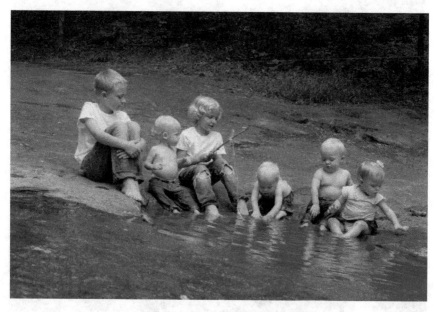

A Moment of Peace with All Six

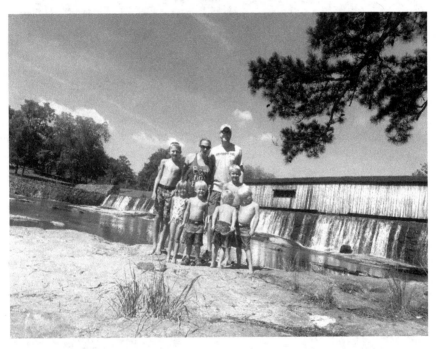

There Is Always One Not Looking at the Camera

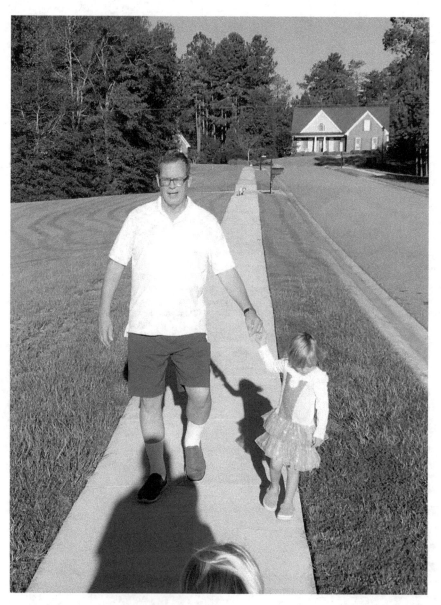

Dad's Last Walk with Bradlee

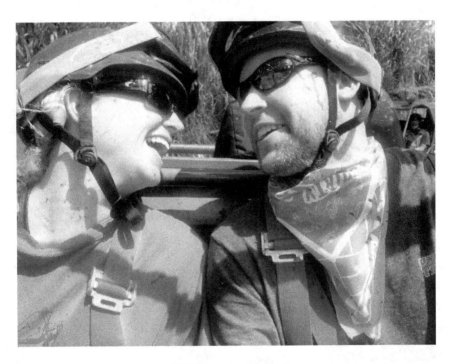

ATV Tour in Hawaii

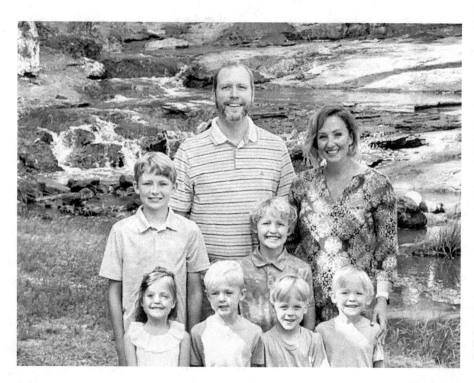

Our Beautiful Chaos

REFERENCES

1. John C. Maxwell, *The 21 Irrefutable Laws of Leadership: Follow Them and People Will Follow You* (Nashville: Thomas Nelson, 2007).

2. *Rocky Balboa.* Directed by Sylvester Stallone. Metro-Goldwyn-Mayer (MGM), Columbia Pictures, Revolution Studios, 2006.

3. Al Capone, accessed August 1, 2020, https://www.goodreads.com/quotes/922378-don-t-mistake-my-kindness-for-weakness-i-am-kind-to.

4. Carly Fiorina, *Find Your Way: Unleash Your Power and Highest Potential.* (Chicago: Tyndale House, 2019).

5. Bonnie Bonadeo, "When Emotions Are High, Intelligence Is Low," May 20, 2013, https://www.modernsalon.com/365006/when-emotions-are-high-intelligence-is-low.

6. Rich Roll, "Susan David, Ph.D., on the Power of Emotional Agility & Why Discomfort Is the Price of Admission to a Meaningful Life," March 25, 2018, https://www.richroll.com/podcast/susan-david-356/.

7. "Stevens-Johnson syndrome/toxic epidermal necrolysis," Genetic and Rare Diseases Information Center (GARD), last updated 10/8/2018, https://rarediseases.info.nih.gov/diseases/7700/stevens-johnson-syndrometoxic-epidermal-necrolysis.

8. Joyce Meyer, July 9, 2018, https://godtv.com/21-inspiring-joyce-meyer-quote/.

9. *Trolls*. Directed by Mike Mitchell. DreamWorks Animation, 2016.

10. "Home." Track #4, *Never Lose Sight*, sixstepsrecords/Sparrow Records, 2016, Album. Chris Tomlin.

11. IULIA-CRISTINA UȚĂ, "The Self-Improvement Industry Is Estimated to Grow to $13.2 billion by 2022," June 27, 2020, http://brandminds.live/the-self-improvement-industry-is-estimated-to-grow-to-13-2-billion-by-2022/.

12. "What Is the Tony Robbins Firewalk?" November 19, 2017, https://tonyrobbinsfirewalk.com/what-is-the-tony-robbins-firewalk/.

ABOUT THE AUTHOR

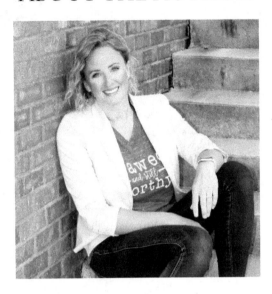

Julianne Kirkland started writing about her journey to becoming a mother of six when she was parenting toddlers and discovered she was pregnant with quadruplets. Her blog *Oh My Quad* eventually reached over 300,000 followers.

An entrepreneur to her core, she grew her salon business even while on bed rest. Today, she dances through mountains of laundry, but when she collapses on the floor to rest, she lets her kids play with the extra skin on her tummy. And unless she's going out on a date night with her hunky hubs, she doesn't actually do her makeup every day. She lets her Instagram filter do it for her.

Today, as a speaker and life coach, Julianne helps ambitious women rise above life's overwhelming obstacles to create their ideal future and manifest abundance through faith. As they elevate their mindset, align with God's calling, and discover his purpose for their lives, they experience powerful life transformation.

Find out more about her transformative coaching program at InspiredLifeMentor.com.